Psychiatry for the Boards

Psychiatry for the Boards

Wen-Hui Cai, M.D., Ph.D.
Senior Resident
Department of Psychiatry
Washington University School of Medicine
St. Louis, Missouri

William W. Wang, M.D., Ph.D.
Senior Resident
Department of Psychiatry
Washington University School of Medicine
St. Louis, Missouri

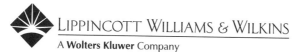

LIPPINCOTT WILLIAMS & WILKINS
A **Wolters Kluwer** Company

Philadelphia · Baltimore · New York · London
Buenos Aires · Hong Kong · Sydney · Tokyo

Acquisitions Editor: Charles W. Mitchell
Developmental Editor: Stacey L. Baze
Production Editor: Emily Lerman
Manufacturing Manager: Chris Rice
Cover Designer: Christine Jenny
Compositor: Lippincott Williams & Wilkins Desktop Division
Printer: Edwards Brothers

© 2002 by **LIPPINCOTT WILLIAMS & WILKINS**
530 Walnut Street
Philadelphia, PA 19106 USA
LWW.com

Printed in the USA

Library of Congress Cataloging-in-Publication Data

Psychiatry for the boards / editors, Wen-Hui Cai, William W. Wang.
   p.; cm.
   Includes index.
   ISBN: 0-7817-4159-9
   1. Psychiatry—Examinations, questions, etc.   I. Cai, Wen-Hui, M.D.   II. Wang, William W.
   [DNLM: 1. Psychiatry—Examination Questions. WM 18.2 P9732 2002]
   RC457.P775 2002
   616.89'0076—dc21   2002072984

10 9 8 7 6 5 4 3 2 1

To Fangru, David, and Mark—
WHC

To Yujia—
WWW

Contents

Introduction

This book is a collection of the most updated, high-yield information to improve your performance in the standard national examinations in clinical psychiatry. These examinations include Psychiatry Resident In-Training Examination (PRITE), the American Board of Psychiatry and Neurology written board examination (Board), and the United States Medical License Examination (USMLE) Steps 2 and 3.

This book is not designed to replace a textbook. It is not intended to be comprehensive. Therefore, it does not offer much simple and basic knowledge. Our primary criterion in selecting the material was its relevance to the PRITE, BOARD, and USMLE examinations. We strove to curtail the content so that this book would be brief yet serve as an effective test preparation tool.

The text is divided into two columns. The left column contains core items and questions. The right column contains corresponding explanations and answers. The right column offers, in italic print, cross-references, mnemonics, and illustrations that we believe particularly helpful. Throughout the book, the most essential information is underlined. Items are written in a variety of formats, including rapid-fire question/answer, brief outline, and short passage. Some information is intentionally repeated in different sections. We have found that variety and repetition are both powerful motivators in sustaining attention and enhancing memorization.

This book was written for psychiatry residents and practicing psychiatrists. This book should also be helpful to senior medical students who are considering a career in psychiatry, and to physicians of other specialties in which questions about mental illness, behavioral problems, and cognitive functions appear in their standard examinations.

We are confident that no other currently available psychiatry review book offers the readers so much carefully selected, test-focused information in such a concise and easy-to-read format. We believe the information in this book will significantly improve your scores on the PRITE, Board, and USMLE examinations in a period of several weeks.

Wen-Hui Cai, M.D., Ph.D.
William W. Wang, M.D., Ph.D.

Chapter 1 Psychological Theories and Behavioral Sciences

What is attachment?

Attachment is the emotional and behavioral dependence of an infant on its primary caregiver. It involves the senses of resources and security.

Attachment develops between the ages of 6 to 8 weeks and 3 years, and lasts for life.

The term "bonding" is often used alternatively for attachment. However, bonding is not associated with resources and security (e.g., a mother feels anxious but does not feel unsafe when she is separated from her infant).

Attachment: Child → Mother

Bonding: Mother → Child

Insecure attachments may be associated with the development of personality disorders.

Attachment theory was developed by John Bowlby.

What is the "strange situation?"

Developed by Mary Ainsworth in the mid-1980s, "strange situation" is a research protocol for assessing an infant's attachment.

What is classical conditioning?

Also called "respondent conditioning," classical conditioning results from the repeated pairing of a neutral (conditioned) stimulus with one that evokes a response (unconditioned stimulus), such that the neutral stimulus eventually comes to evoke the response.

Example: A dog salivated when it had food in its mouth, saw the food, smelled the food, or even when it heard the footsteps of a person coming to feed the dog.

Food: Unconditioned stimulus (UCS).

Food → salivation: Unconditioned response (UCR).

Footsteps: Conditioned stimulus (CS).

Footstep → salivation: Conditioned response (CR).

The concept of classical conditioning was developed by Ivan Pavlov.

In classical conditioning theory, what are extinction, generalization, and discrimination?

Extinction: When a CS is repeated without being paired with its UCS, the CR gradually weakens and eventually disappears. However, the UCR does not become extinct.

Generalization: The transferring of a CS from one stimulus to another. A dog may respond to the footsteps of people other than its feeder, or even to noises other than footsteps. Transference during psychotherapy was explained as stimulus generalization.

Discrimination: Recognizing and responding to differences between similar stimuli. A smart dog knows when its feeder is coming.

How does one maintain a behavior so that it is resistant to extinction?

Give the positive reinforcement intermittently, and in a variable-ratio schedule.

Mechanism of extinction applied to substance-related disorders:

CS (conditioned stimulus): Environment associated with craving.

UCS (unconditioned stimulus): Drug.

CR (conditioned response): Craving.

CR was established with repeated exposure to a paired UCS and CS. When the patient is repeatedly exposed to an unpaired CS (i.e., when a UCS is not available), the craving may finally become extinct.

What is operant conditioning?

It is a form of learning in which behavioral frequency is altered through the application of positive and negative consequences. Operant conditioning is also known as "instrumental conditioning."

Example: A dog receives food only when it responds correctly by pressing a lever.

Food: Reinforcing stimulus.

Lever: Operant.

The concept of operant conditioning was developed by B.F. Skinner.

Reinforcement.

Positive reinforcement: Increases the probability that a response will recur.

Negative reinforcement: Leads to the removal of a response.

Variable-interval schedule: Reinforcement occurs at variable intervals.

State-dependent learning.

Recall of information is facilitated by the same environment in which the information was first acquired.

One may do better in an examination by wearing the same earplugs as worn when studying for the examination.

According to Eric Erikson, what is the developmental task between the ages of 40 and 60?

This stage is the seventh stage in Erikson's life-cycle theory. Adults at this stage must choose between generativity and stagnation (cessation of growth, becoming stale). A successful choice in the developmental task is generativity, that is, becoming useful to society through behaviors that protect future generations.

Eric Erikson's eight stages of the life cycle are:

1. *Basic trust versus basic mistrust (0 to 1 years).*
2. *Autonomy versus shame and doubt (1 to 3 years).*
3. *Initiative versus guilt (3 to 5 years).*
4. *Industry versus inferiority (6 to 11 years).*
5. *Identity versus role confusion (11 to 20 years).*
6. *Intimacy versus self-absorption or isolation (21 to 40 years).*
7. *Generativity versus stagnation (40 to 65 years).*
8. *Integrity versus despair and isolation (65 years and older).*

What are characteristic features of Eric Erikson's stage of industry versus inferiority? To which of Sigmund Freud's stages of psychosexual development does this stage correspond?

In Erikson's stage of industry versus inferiority (6 to 11 years), children are busy building, creating, and accomplishing. They are able <u>to set up clubs with complicated rules and rituals.</u> They also face the danger of a sense of inadequacy and inferiority. This stage corresponds to Freud's latency stage (5 to 12 years).

What is sublimation?

Sublimation is a defense mechanism through which unhealthy or unacceptable drives and affects are transformed into healthy and creative behavior.

What is conventional morality?

Conventional morality is one of the major levels of morality development. Integrating Jean Piaget's cognitive development theory, Lawrence Kohlberg described three major levels of morality:

1. Preconventional: To obey and to avoid punishment.
2. Conventional: To gain approval from others, especially peers.
3. Principle: To comply with ethical principles.

What are the principal concepts in Carol Gilligan's model of morality?

Carol Gilligan believes that there are alternate pathways to the same moral pinnacle. She proposed that girls have a greater sense of connection and concern with relationships than with rules (i.e., that girls rely on intuitive sense in decision making).

According to modern psychodynamic theory, what factors are the most important in the formation of adult personality?

The most important factors are:

1. Inherited traits.
2. Environment.
3. Experiences of infancy and childhood.

What is "learned helplessness?"

It is an animal model of depression. After a period of intermittent electric shocks from which there is no possible escape, the animal gave up further attempts to escape from the shocks.

The concept of learned helplessness was developed by Martin Seligman and is a well-recognized model of an experimental depressive disorder. The apparent cessation of efforts to escape from shock becomes generalized to other situations, and eventually the animal always becomes helpless and apathetic.

Primary process versus secondary process.

According to Sigmund Freud, primary-process thinking is the primitive form of cognitive activity that is motivated by the pleasure principle.

Primary-process thinking is revised by the ego to become coherent, mature, and rational. This revision is called the secondary process or secondary revision, and is guided by <u>the reality principle.</u>

What is anal fixation? What personality disorder has its development associated with anal fixation?

According to classic psychoanalytic theory, anal fixation is a form of regression in response to <u>castration anxiety encountered in the oedipal phase.</u> Anally fixated persons are viewed as victims of a harsh and <u>unlenient superego.</u>

The character pattern of anal fixation includes excessive orderliness, <u>perseverance, emotional constriction, a tendency to intellectualize, indecisiveness, procrastination,</u> and stubbornness. All of these features are characteristic <u>for obsessive–compulsive personality disorder.</u>

The stages of psychosexual development set forth in Sigmund Freud's theory are:

1. *Oral (birth to 18 months).*
2. *Anal (1 to 3 years).*
3. *Phallic (Oedipal, 3 to 5 years).*
4. *Latency (5 to 12 years).*
5. *Genital (12 years to adulthood).*

What is psychic determinism?

One of the principal beliefs of psychoanalysis is that behavior has meaning. A particular behavior is determined by "psychic" motivation in the form of <u>unconscious drives,</u>

defenses, object relationships, and self-disturbances. A central feature of psychic determinism is that childhood experiences are repeated throughout life.

On the basis of Salvador Minuchin's theory of family interactions, explain the phenomenon of a mother constantly staying with her ill son and calling his disease "our disease."

Salvador Minuchin was one of the early conceptualists of the family system, and the originator of structural family therapy.

Structural family therapy focuses on the current organization (structure) of a family.

Analysis of interactions (between family members, in therapeutic sessions) allows the therapist to clarify how the family's organization influences (promotes or inhibits) task performance, especially child-rearing.

The therapist promotes those interactions that introduce greater flexibility, alternative patterns and structures, and more effective task performance.

Enmeshment (ineffective closeness) and disengagement (excessive distance), as well as rapid fluctuations between interactional extremes, are manifestations of dysfunctional family relationships.

Other core concepts of Minuchin's theory include boundaries, hierarchies, coalitions, alliances, and complementarity.

The case described above, of the mother remaining with her ill son, is a typical case of <u>enmeshment.</u>

Minuchin's form of family therapy was developed to address child and adolescent emotional and behavioral problems, and is particularly effective in such situations. It is arguably the most influential form of family therapy.

What did Stephen Suomi's studies of the total isolation of infant monkeys imply?

These studies implied that <u>"therapist" monkeys could help socialize infants.</u>

In 1972, Stephen Suomi demonstrated that monkey isolates could be rehabilitated if they were exposed to monkeys that promote physical contact without threatening the isolates with aggression or overly complex play interactions. These monkeys were called therapist monkeys. To fill such a therapeutic role, Suomi chose young normal monkeys that played gently with the isolates and would approach and cling to them. Within 2 weeks, the isolates were reciprocating the social contact, and their incidence of abnormal self-directed behaviors began to decline significantly. By the end of a

6-month treatment period, the isolates were actively initiating play bouts with both the therapist monkeys and each other, and most of their self-directed behaviors had disappeared. Two years later, the isolates' improved behavior had not regressed.

Chapter 2 Psychometric and Neuropsychological Testing

What is the best psychological test to use for assessing possible malingering?

The Minnesota Multiphasic Personality Inventory (MMPI).

What are the best tests with which to assess executive function?

Trail-making tests (e.g., the patient is requested to give sequentially alternative numbers and letters: 1-Z-2-Y-3-X...). These tests require rapid and efficient visual–motor integration, attention, and cognitive sequencing.

Card-sorting tests (e.g., Wisconsin Card Sorting Test [WCST]).

What is Bender Gestalt Test?

Also known as the Bender Visual–Motor Gestalt Test, the Bender Gestalt Test is a psychological test to assess visuomotor integration and visual construction. Originally designed to measure maturational levels in children, the test may suggest some deficiency in construction ability. Signs of brain damage on the Bender Gestalt Test include visual neglect, rotation of designs, perseveration, and distorted designs.

What should a psychiatrist bear in mind when drawing inferences from computerized interpretations of the MMPI-II?

The accuracy of the interpretive statements varies among interpretive services.

Which psychiatric instrument is most useful for distinguishing an episodic psychiatric disorder from lifelong personality traits in an adult?

The Structured Clinical Interview from the *Diagnostic and Statistical Manual of Mental Disorders, Fourth Revision* (DSM-IV).

What are the uses of each following neuropsychological tests?

1. Thematic Apperception Test (TAT).
2. Brief Psychiatric Rating Scale (BPRS).
3. Millon Clinical Multiaxial Inventory-II.
4. Halstead–Reitan Neuropsychological Battery.
5. MMPI-II.

Developed by Murray and Morgan, the <u>TAT</u> is used to test <u>normal personality</u> by having a person tell a story after viewing each of a series of ambiguous pictures showing one or more people in various settings.

The <u>BPRS</u> is one of several psychometric instruments used to assess for schizophrenia and psychoses.

The <u>Millon Clinical Multiaxial Inventory-II</u> measures personality styles, expressed concerns, and behavioral correlates. There is also a Millon Adolescent Personality Inventory.

The <u>Halstead–Reitan Neuropsychological Battery</u> is used to examine for the location and effects of specific brain lesions. It includes 10 tests, respectively, for category, tactile performance, perception of rhythm, finger-oscillation, perception of speech-sounds, trail-making, perception of critical flicker frequency, time sense, aphasia screening, and sensory-perceptual function. It can be used <u>to differentiate among early dementia, mild delirium, and depression.</u>

<u>The MMPI-II</u> is a self-report inventory that is the most widely used and most thoroughly researched objective instrument for personality assessment. It contains more than 500 statements and gives scores on 10 standard clinical scales. It is used <u>to identify major areas of psychopathologic functioning.</u>

What is the purpose of projective testing?

<u>To detect the presence of subtle psychotic thought processes</u> and bizarre ideation.

Common projective tests include the:

Rorschach Test.
TAT.
Sentence Completion Test.
Word-Association Technique.
Draw-a-person test.

The MMPI is not a projective test.

What does the WCST assess?

Abstract reasoning and flexibility in problem solving.

A patient scores very low in Wechsler Adult Intelligence Scale, Revised (WAIS-R) subtests for picture arrangement and block design as compared to other subtests. What does this result suggest?

A lesion in the nondominant hemisphere.

What does the comprehension subtest of the WAIS measure?

It measures the ability to abstract and adhere to social conventions.

Besides malingering, what might be the reason for an inaccurate result of Mini-Mental Status Examination?

A false-negative result may occur in patients with restricted deficits.

Chapter 3 Epidemiology, Biostatistics, and Social Psychiatry

What is a cohort study?

A cohort study is a study that follows a group of subjects chosen from <u>a well-defined population</u> over an <u>extended period.</u> It is a form of prospective study.

Cohort study (also known as a follow-up study): a group of individuals (cohort) is defined on the basis of having or lacking exposure to a suspected risk factor for a disease, and is followed for an extended period.

Case–Control study: subjects are selected on the basis of whether they do or do not have the particular disease being studied.

Descriptive studies (including correlation studies, case reports or case series, and cross-sectional surveys): describe patterns of disease occurrence in relation to selected variables (e.g., person, place, and time).

Intervention study: the investigator controls the allocation of subjects to different comparison groups and regulates the experimental conditions for each group.

What research design is necessary to establish a causal inference for an observed effect?	A control group study.
Construct validity.	Construct validity is the ability of a test to measure <u>what it is designed to assess.</u>
Reliability.	Reliability is the repeatability of the finding of an assessment instrument.
What is the most important factor in deciding the validity of a worker's compensation case?	A <u>causal link</u> between an occurrence at work and subsequent illness.
What do the sensitivity and specificity of a test measure?	Sensitivity measures the ability of a test to identify <u>true-positive</u> cases. Specificity measures the ability of a test to identify <u>true-negative</u> cases.
What is sensitivity?	The proportion of positive test results among the test group of individuals who actually have a particular condition.
Racial differences in pharmacokinetics.	Racial differences in pharmacokinetics are usually based on differences in liver enzymes. For example, <u>lithium</u> is not metabolized in the liver, there are therefore few racial differences in its metabolism.

Regression analysis.	A procedure for predicting the value or behavior of one variable (the dependent variable) on the basis of the value or behavior of another variable (the independent variable). For example, one may predict a student's performance in college (X) on the basis of the student's score on a scholastic aptitude test (Y).
	Y is a known value, and is the independent variable.
	X is an unknown value but is somehow dependent upon Y, and is therefore the dependent variable.
In recent years, the suicide rate has increased in which population group?	Since 1960, suicide has increased dramatically among <u>adolescents.</u>
What is the best factor for predicting suicide?	The best factor for predicting suicide is <u>the subject's past suicidal behavior.</u>
What is the "drift hypothesis?"	The drift hypothesis states that disabling conditions tend to cause downward social mobility. This hypothesis offered one of the explanations for the early finding that schizophrenia and other mental disorders were more prevalent among people of low socio-economic status.

What factors have caused an increased need for geriatric long-term mental health care?

The <u>increase in size of the geriatric population</u> and the <u>lack of family supports</u> are two important factors in the increased need for geriatric long-term mental health care.

What factors are associated with the seeking of psychiatric help?

Gender, social class, and education.

Gender: More women than men seek psychiatric help.

Social class: People of higher social class are more likely to use psychiatric services.

Education: Higher education is associated with more frequent use of psychiatric services.

What is the most common method for completed suicide among adolescents?

Use of a gun.

What type of prevention is demonstrated by abstinence from alcohol during pregnancy?

<u>Primary prevention.</u>

Primary prevention: preventing the onset of a disease and thereby reducing its incidence by eliminating the causative agents, reducing risk factors, enhancing host resistance, and interfering with transmission of the disease.

Secondary prevention: early identification and prompt treatment of an illness, with the goal of reducing its prevalence by reducing its duration.

Tertiary prevention: reducing the prevalence of residual defects and disabilities caused by an illness; this enables those with chronic mental illnesses to reach the highest feasible level of function.

Give an example of tertiary prevention.

Enabling persons with severe, persistent mental illness to reach their highest level of functioning.

What type of prevention is involved in helping schizophrenia patients to attain their maximal level of functioning?

Tertiary prevention.

Prevalence versus incidence

Prevalence is the proportion of individuals with <u>existing disease</u> at a point in time (point prevalence) or during a period of time (period prevalence).

Incidence is the proportion of individuals developing <u>new disease</u> during a period of time.

Prevalence refers to all persons who are diseased.

Incidence refers only to new cases.

There is no such thing as "point incidence."

How should one select a statistical test for evaluating the significance of a finding? (It is very easy to earn extra points here, so be patient in reading the long passage that follows.)

Step one: Know the type of data to be tested. The appropriate choice of a statistical test depends upon the type of data to which it is to be applied.

There are four types of data: Nominal, ordinal, interval, and ratio.

Nominal data are groups with no ordering (e.g., 25 males, 171 treatment respondents, 6 counties). Nominal data cannot be used to generate means and standard deviations.

Ordinal data are groups in rank order (e.g., class standing, personal preferences).

Interval data are data measured on a scale of equal intervals (e.g., temperature, height, dosage, weight). Interval data can be used to generate means and standard deviations.

A ratio is a comparison between interval data and a true or zero point (e.g., suicide rate, disease prevalence).

Nominal and interval data are frequently tested in PRITE and the Board. For statistical purposes, ratio data are treated like interval data. Ordinal data are rarely used.

Step two: Choose the right test for the type of data to be tested.

Five types of statistical tests are commonly used in psychiatric research: the <u>T-test, Chi-square test, analysis of variance (ANOVA), Pearson's coefficient correlation, and regression.</u>

If only interval data are being used, Pearson's coefficient correlation (to reveal a linear association) or regression analysis (to reveal a nonlinear nature of the relationship) should be applied.

If only nominal data are being used, the Chi-square test should be applied.

If combined interval and nominal data are being used, and two groups of data are being compared, the T-test should be used. If more than two groups of data are being compared, ANOVA should be used.

What is meta-analysis?

Meta-analysis is a procedure that combines results from a number of similarly designed studies to estimate the effect of a variable by incorporating the information provided by all the studies.

What psychiatric illness is most frequently related to completed suicide?	Major depression.
What is standard deviation?	The degree of spread of values around the mean.
What does a *p* value of 0.05 mean?	The probability of obtaining the result by chance alone is 1:20 (5%).
Based on epidemiologic studies (National Institute of Mental Health Epidemiological Catchment Area Study), what mental illness is more likely in a male population?	<u>Substance Abuse.</u> *What mental illnesses are more likely in a female population?* *Major depression, borderline personality, panic disorder.* *What mental illnesses are not favored in populations of either gender?* *Schizophrenia and bipolar I affective disorder.*
What is the most common cause of death among African–American male youths?	Homicide.
What is the most frequently reported child abuse in the United States?	Child neglect.

National Alliance for the Mentally Ill.	Members: Families and relatives of patients. Goal: To improve patient services and research.
Psychiatric service models.	Assertive community treatment: active outreach to patients. Traditional social work: helps patients connect to existing services.
What is reparative therapy? What is the standpoint of the American Psychiatric Association (APA) on this issue?	A variety of psychotherapeutic approaches were developed from the 1950s to 1970s to "repair" the sexual orientation of homosexual persons. Since the 1970s, the APA has held the position that homosexuality is a nonpathologic human potential rather than a disorder. No existing evidence supports or advises reparative therapy for it.
What is the most common mistaken diagnosis that psychiatrists make in African–American patients who have major depression or bipolar disorder?	Schizophrenia.

What is the most characteristic manifestation of depression in Chinese–American patients, and how should it be approached?

Chinese–American patients with depression tend to have many somatic complaints, and should be approached with direct questions about mood symptoms.

What do Japanese–American female patients commonly do to make their stories discrepant from collateral information when presenting with a depressive history?

They seek to minimize their distress in front of an authority figure.

What does it mean when a third-party payer says that it offers parity in mental health treatment?

Parity in this case means that mental health services are covered on a par with other health services.

What did the National Institute of Mental Health Epidemiological Catchment Area study indicate about depression in younger and older cohorts?

It showed that <u>depression now occurs at an earlier age than it previously did, and at an increased rate as compared with the past.</u>

Chapter 4   Neuroscience

What are the major inhibitory neurotransmitters?

<u>γ-Aminobutyric acid (GABA)</u> and glycine.

Neurotransmitters:

Excitatory: Glutamate.

Inhibitory: GABA and glycine.

Which cerebral lobes are considered to be associated with executive functioning?

The frontal lobes.

What are the locations of cell bodies that produce major neurotransmitters?

1. Serotonin; two locations:
   a. <u>Raphe nuclei</u> (upper pons and midbrain).
   b. Caudal locus ceruleus (to a lesser extent).
2. Dopamine; three locations:
   a. Substantia nigra (<u>nigrostriatal pathway,</u> associated with extrapyramidal syndrome).
   b. Ventral tegmental area (VTA, mesolimbic–mesocortical pathway, associated with antipsychotic effects and reward system).
   c. Hypothalamus, including the arcuate and periventricular nuclei (tuberoinfundibular pathway, associated with prolactin regulation).

3. Norepinephrine: <u>Locus caeruleus</u> (pons).

The mesolimbic–mesocortical dopamine pathway is actually a combination of two pathways that may be heavily involved in the symptomatology of schizophrenia:

Mesolimbic pathway: positive symptoms.

Mesocortical pathway: negative symptoms.

What is the endocrinologic effect of dopamine?

Dopamine inhibits the release of prolactin (tuberoinfundibular pathway).

What is the reward system?

A neuropsychological system associated with feelings of reward and satisfaction. It is hypothesized as being associated with the mesolimbic–mesocortical dopamine pathway. This is thought to be the primary neurophysiologic mechanism of addiction.

Which neurotransmitters influence aggressive behavior?

Induction of aggression: Dopamine.

Inhibition of aggression: Norepinephrine, serotonin, GABA.

The levels of <u>5-hydroxyindoleacetic acid (5-HIAA)</u> (the major serotonin metabolite) in cerebrospinal fluid (CSF) *inversely* correlate with the frequency of aggression.

What is the significance of a low 5-HIAA level in CSF?

It is associated with aggressive behavior and with suicide by violent methods.

What is the function of GABA receptors?

They are functionally related to chloride channels that are regulated by GABA and other ligands. When GABA binds to its receptors, the chloride channels open, allowing more chloride influx into the cell, and therefore an increase in membrane polarization. Benzodiazepines bind to specific sites on GABA receptors and facilitate the effects of GABA (i.e., they increase the affinity of the GABA receptors for GABA).

What is excitotoxicity?

A hypothesis states that excessive stimulation of glutamate receptors may lead to prolonged high intraneuronal concentrations of calcium and nitric oxide. Such conditions activate many proteases and finally destroy the neuron.

Excitatory neurotransmitter: Glutamate.

Inhibitory neurotransmitters: GABA and glycine.

Summary of characteristics of dopamine receptors.

1. All dopamine receptors are membrane-anchored receptors.
2. All dopamine receptors are G-protein linked.
3. Major subtypes of dopamine receptors are D1, D2, D3, D4, and D5.
4. Activation of <u>D1 and D5 results in an increase of cyclic adenosine monophosphate (cAMP).</u> Activation of D2–D4 receptors results in a decrease of cAMP. Activation of D2 receptors is also associated with increased potassium conductance.

What genetic disorders are associated with unstable triplet (trinucleotide) repeat sequences?

<u>Huntington's disease, Fragile X syndrome, myotonic dystrophy,</u> spinobulbar muscular atrophy, spinocerebellar ataxia type 1, and Machado–Joseph disease.

What is the major neuroimaging finding in attention-deficit/hyperactivity disorder?

Decreased metabolism in the frontal lobes.

Which neurotransmitters are and which are not associated with anxiety?

Neurotransmitters associated with anxiety:

Norepinephrine, serotonin, and GABA.

Neurotransmitters not associated with anxiety:

Dopamine, glutamate, histamine, a cetylcholine.

Chapter 5 Psychiatric Interview, Symptomatology, and Diagnosis

What is delusion?

It is fixed, false belief that is <u>unreal, idiosyncratic, and not accepted by other members of the same subcultural background.</u>

What was the dominant intellectual perspective in psychiatry in the 19th century throughout Europe and the United States?

Biological psychiatry.

What is circumstantiality?

It is a patient's discussion of unnecessary details and inappropriate thoughts before communicating a central idea. The patient should ultimately be able to reach the key point of the discussion.

Inability of the patient to reach the central point of a discussion even with sufficient time is called tangentiality.

What symptoms are associated with a dissociative phenomenon?

<u>Derealization,</u> depersonalization, dissociative amnesia, and fugue.

What is dissociation?	It is a splitting away of thoughts, feelings, or behaviors from conscious awareness.
What is the least clinically significant form of disorientation?	<u>Disorientation to day or date.</u> (It is so common that it happens in 60% of normal people.)
What should be accomplished during the initial assessment for psychodynamic psychotherapy?	An initial treatment plan, a mental-status assessment, a descriptive psychiatric diagnosis, and an initial psychodynamic formulation.
What is channeling?	Channeling is a meditative or trancelike state with the purpose of conveying messages from a spiritual guide. Channeling is often introduced as a culturally mediated, specific response to distress. It is considered a <u>nonpathologic form of dissociation.</u>
What is the serotonin syndrome?	It is the cluster of symptoms of <u>restlessness, myoclonus, hyperreflexia, diaphoresis, shivering, tremor, and confusion,</u> which usually follows the use of a monoamine oxidase inhibitor too soon after the failure of a tricyclic antidepressant or serotonin-specific reuptake inhibitor to let TCA or SSRI totally diminish from the body.
What is compulsion?	Repetitive, stereotyped behavior in which <u>the patient recognizes the irrationality of the behavior.</u>

What is Capgras' syndrome?	The belief that an impostor has replaced a significant other (usually a family member).
What is Ganser syndrome?	The production of approximate answers (*vorbeireden*) to questions. This may be a manifestation of malingering, a state of confusion, or a disinhibition syndrome.
	The term vorbeireden, circumlocution and failure to reach the central idea of a discussion, is not now popularly used in the psychiatric literature. Vorbeireden was sometimes used as an equivalent term to tangentiality.
What is alexithymia?	Difficulty in recognizing and describing one's emotions.
Is hallucination a part of the content of thought (COT)?	No. Inclusion of hallucination in COT is a popular mistake. Hallucination is a false sensory perception.
Between which two editions of the *Diagnostic and Statistical Manual of Mental Disorders* (DSM) did the diagnostic principle and approach to psychiatric illness undergo a major revision?	From DSM-II to DSM-III, in which a new medical model, with an evidence-based, research-driven approach replaced the psychodynamic theory-dominated model.

How is genuine auditory hallucination differentiated from malingering?

Thorough and prolonged examination and observation, plus good collateral information, may be the best way to differentiate the two. Reported characteristics of malingered auditory hallucination include <u>the lack of a strategy to diminish the hallucinated voices,</u> and reported use of stilted language by the voices (e.g., "Go commit a sex offense").

Chapter 6 Dementia and Delirium

What is the first step in the treatment of delirium?

Protecting the patient from unintentional harm.

What are the frontal lobe syndromes?

A variety of psychiatric symptoms that result from lesions in a frontal lobe. The locations of these lesions, and their effects, are as follows:

Orbitofrontal: Disinhibition, impulsiveness. Patients may become <u>profane, irascible, and irresponsible.</u>

Medial frontal: Apathy.

Left frontal: Depression.

Right frontal: Mania.

A well-educated and conscientious man who becomes greedy, selfish, and irritable may have a tumor in a frontal lobe.

What is the pharmacologic treatment for Alzheimer's disease, and by what mechanisms does it act?

Treatment: Cholinesterase inhibitors, which <u>block the catabolism of acetylcholine, and therefore boost central acetylcholine levels,</u> in the central nervous system. These drugs include donepezil, tacrine, and rivastigmine.

What is perseveration?

A disturbance in form of thought. This symptom is often associated with cognitive disorders. The patient exhibits a persisting response to a previous stimulus after a new stimulus has been presented. For example, the patient may draw a circle when asked to do so, but continues to draw circles when asked to draw squares.

What disorder in early life has pathologic changes similar to those of Alzheimer's disease?

<u>Down's syndrome.</u>

Both Alzheimer's disease and Down's syndrome are associated with defects in chromosome 21. Persons with Down's syndrome who survive into early adulthood may present with histopathologic changes that are typical in Alzheimer's disease (senile plaques and neurofibrillary tangles).

There is also a clear <u>familial association</u> of Alzheimer's disease with Down's syndrome.

What are the clinical manifestations of multi-infarct dementia?

1. <u>Stepwise progression</u> of deficits.
2. Pseudobulbar palsy.
3. <u>Focal</u> sensorimotor abnormalities.

What are the neuroimaging findings in Alzheimer's disease?

Neuroimaging does not yet have a clear role in the diagnosis of Alzheimer's disease. Reported findings in the disease include hypometabolism and atrophy in the frontal, parietal, and temporal lobes.

What is delirium?

It is a disturbance of consciousness, with changes in attention, cognition (which includes memory, especially short-term recent memory; orientation; and language), and perception (marked by hallucinations, behavioral changes, and labile affect). Delirium usually develops over a short period and tends to fluctuate during the course of the day.

What electroencephalographic feature may appear in delirium?

Generalized slow (theta and delta) activity, and sometimes focal areas of hyperactivity.

Chapter 7   Substance-Related Disorders

What are the purposes of pharmacologic treatment for alcoholism, and what agents are used to achieve them?

To reduce craving: Opioid antagonists (<u>naltrexone, nalmefene</u>), serotonin-specific reuptake inhibitors (<u>fluoxetine, citalopram</u>), lithium, bromocriptine.

Withdrawal: <u>Benzodiazepines.</u>

Adverse conditioning: <u>Disulfiram.</u>

What is the characteristic electrophysiologic finding in alcoholic neuropathy?

Attenuated sensory and motor amplitudes.

What abnormalities in hepatic function tests are most likely to be associated with chronic alcohol abuse?

1. The <u>γ-glutamyl transferase</u> level is elevated in 80% of patients.
2. Serum glutamic oxaloacetic transaminase (SGOT) and serum glutamic pyruvic transaminase (SGPT) are both elevated, but SGOT is higher than SGPT.
3. Mean corpuscular volume is increased in 60% of patients.

SG<u>O</u>T is higher with EtO̲H.

What is idiosyncratic alcohol intoxication?

It is a severe behavioral syndrome that develops rapidly after a person consumes <u>a small amount</u> of alcohol that would have minimal behavioral effects on most people.

The patient can be confused and disoriented, and can have illusions, transitory delusions, and visual hallucinations, as well as displaying <u>labile affect, slurred speech, and intoxicated behavior,</u> with greatly increased psychomotor activity and impulsive, aggressive behavior that may be dangerous. The <u>serum alcohol level</u> is usually low (e.g., <u>under 50 ng/dL</u>).

This syndrome usually occurs in persons with high levels of anxiety or of advancing age, or with sedative-hypnotic drug use and a feeling of fatigue. The behavior tends to be atypical. This diagnosis is still debatable, but is important in the forensic arena.

Which subtype of anxiety disorder is most commonly associated with alcohol-related disorder?

Panic disorder.

What psychotic symptoms may present with alcohol withdrawal? What treatment is indicated?

Alcohol withdrawal may typically present with transient visual, tactile, or auditory <u>hallucinations.</u>

The first-choice treatment is a <u>benzodiazepine.</u> Low-dose, short treatment with antipsychotic agents may be needed.

What medication decreases the incidence of relapse in alcohol-dependent patients?

Naltrexone, but not disulfiram.

What are the mechanisms of action of disulfiram in reducing alcohol intake?

Disulfiram inhibits the alcohol-degrading enzyme acetaldehyde dehydrogenase, and therefore raises acetaldehyde levels in the blood and tissues. It also inhibits dopamine β-hydroxylase.

Its clinical effects last for up to 2 weeks after the last dose.

What are some characteristics of women with alcoholism?

Women with alcoholism are more likely to have it begin at a later age, to have mood disorder, and to use drugs.

What research data support the concept of hereditary factors in alcoholism?

Hereditary grounds for alcoholism were supported by studies of adopted siblings. The famous Danish adoption studies of familial determinants of alcoholism demonstrated that biologic sons of alcoholic individuals were at higher risk of alcoholism than were biologic sons of nonalcoholic individuals.

What is the mission of Al-Anon?

To help relatives cope with an alcoholic's drinking problems.

What drugs could be used to treat a patient who is in alcohol withdrawal who has impaired liver function?

Oxazepam (Serax), lorazepam (Ativan), and temazepam (Restoril), because they do not have intermediate metabolic products that require further metabolism by the liver.

TOL—Tolerated by Our Liver.

What is CAGE questionnaire?

A questionnaire used to screen patients for alcoholism. Its components have the meanings provided below:

Cut: Have you ever felt you should cut down on your drinking?

Annoyed: Have people annoyed you by criticizing your drinking?

Guilt: Have you ever felt guilty about your drinking?

Eye-opener: Have you ever had a drink first thing in the morning to steady your nerves or to get rid of a hangover?

What is delirium tremens (DT)?

A severe alcohol withdrawal syndrome. It constitutes a medical emergency, and if untreated has a high mortality rate (20%).

DT usually occurs within 1 week after a cessation of drinking. It has all the features of delirium. Other symptoms include:

1. Autonomic hyperactivity: Tachycardia, diaphoresis, fever, anxiety, insomnia, and hypertension.
2. A coarse tremor is common.
3. Seizures may occur early in the course of DT.

What is the substance most commonly abused by adolescents?

Alcohol.

The substance most commonly abused by the general population is nicotine.

What is the treatment for Wernicke's syndrome?

Give IV thiamin first! Giving glucose without first replenishing thiamin may exhaust the body's remaining thiamin and worsen the patient's condition.

What is Wernicke–Korsakoff syndrome?

A persisting, alcohol-induced amnestic disorder.

Wernicke's syndrome (also called alcoholic encephalopathy) is a condition of acute onset and is completely reversible.

Korsakoff's syndrome is chronic, and only 20% of patients may recover.

Symptoms of Wernicke's syndrome are:

- Ataxia.
- Confusion.
- Ophthalmoplegia (horizontal nystagmus, paralysis of the abducens, disconjugate eye movements, and gaze palsy).

Pathophysiology: Thiamine deficiency.

Horizontal nystagmus may also appear in phencyclidine intoxication, opioid withdrawal, and eighth-nerve (CN VIII) impairment.

What are the maximum lengths of time for which cocaine metabolites and alcohol can be detected?

Cocaine metabolites: 2 to 4 days.

Alcohol: 7 to 12 hours.

What beverage has the highest concentration of caffeine?

Concentrations of caffeine in the following beverages are in the order shown, from highest to lowest:

Dark chocolate.

Brewed coffee.

Instant coffee.

Tea (leaf or bagged).

Caffeinated soda.

What are the clinical features of cocaine intoxication?

1. Mental: <u>Euphoria,</u> hypervigilance, agitation or psychomotor retardation, <u>hallucinations.</u>
2. Cardiac: <u>Tachycardia,</u> bradycardia, high or low blood pressure, arrhythmia.
3. Other: <u>Pupillary dilation,</u> perspiration or chills, nausea, or vomiting.

<u>Pupillary dilation:</u> <u>C</u>ocaine, lysergic acid diethylamide (LSD), <u>A</u>mphetamine intoxication, or <u>O</u>pioid withdrawal. (Drink COLA, dilate pupils.)

How does cocaine work in the central nervous system?

Cocaine is a competitive blocker of the <u>dopamine transporter.</u> It inhibits dopamine reuptake and increases activation of dopaminergic pathways. It is sometimes called a dopamine agonist.

What is the medical complication commonly associated with cocaine abuse?

Myocardial infarction.

When does cocaine withdrawal occur?

Cocaine withdrawal occurs within hours to days after heavy cocaine use. It is characterized by <u>dysphoria, increased appetite, fatigue,</u> psychomotor retardation or <u>agitation</u>, and sleep abnormalities (dreams, insomnia or hypersomnia).

Vivid, unpleasant dreams occur upon withdrawal from cocaine or amphetamine.

What are the clinical features of LSD intoxication?

1. Behavioral changes: Fear, anxiety, paranoid ideation, impaired judgment.
2. Perceptual changes: Perceptual changes in full wakefulness, depersonalization, derealization, illusions/hallucinations, and synesthesias.
3. Other: Pupillary dilation.

Synesthesia: A sensation or hallucination caused by another sensation.

Pupillary dilation: Cocaine, LSD, Amphetamine intoxication, or Opioid withdrawal. (Drink COLA, dilate pupils.)

What is the mechanism of action of LSD?

LSD is a partial agonist at postsynaptic serotonin receptors.

What is the most popular addictive substance in the United States?

The most popular addictive substance is nicotine.

Among all the abused substances, nicotine addiction contributes most to premature death and disability, and is associated with the highest annual mortality.

What pharmacologic treatment is available for nicotine dependence?

Bupropion (Zyban).

What are common opioid receptor ligands of the opioids?

Agonist: Methadone.

Antagonist: Naltrexone, naloxone, and nalmefene.

Agonist–antagonist: Buprenorphine.

Naloxone and nalmefene: Rapid onset, intravenous (IV) use.

Naltrexone: Slower onset. Used in preventing relapse of alcoholism.

What are the mechanisms of action of opioids?

Opioids specifically bind μ, κ, δ, and probably other types of opioid receptors.

Opioids also have significant effects on the dopaminergic and noradrenergic systems.

Propranolol can potentiate opioid-withdrawal symptoms.

Opium: *The dried, condensed juice of a poppy,* Papaver somniferum.

Opiate: "From opium." Extracts or derivatives of opium.

Opioid: "Opium-like." Includes opiates (alkaloids; e.g., morphine) and endogenous opioids (peptides; e.g., endorphin). "Opioid" is more inclusive and is the preferred term.

What are the symptoms of opioid intoxication and withdrawal, and how are these conditions treated?

1. Opioid-withdrawal symptoms are <u>disorientation, confusion, dysphoric mood, vertical nystagmus, increased muscle tone, mildly enlarged pupils,</u> increased blood pressure and heart rate, <u>marked diaphoresis, piloerection, lacrimation</u> (or rhinorrhea), <u>salivation,</u> nausea or vomiting, diarrhea, yawning, fever, and insomnia.

2. Opioid intoxication symptoms are pupillary constriction with drowsiness or coma, slurred speech, impairment of attention or memory, and <u>pulmonary edema</u> from central respiratory inhibition.

The pupils can be dilated from a severe opioid overdose, as a result of anoxia.

3. Treatment of withdrawal consists of giving <u>clonidine</u> or methadone.
4. Treatment of intoxication consists of giving <u>naloxone</u> at 0.4 mg IV for respiratory depression or <u>stupor.</u>

What should be done first to an opioid-intoxicated patient in the emergency room setting?

Ensure airway support and adequate ventilation. (ABC first!)

What is used to evaluate residual physical dependence in an opioid-dependent patient?

Naloxone.

What are the clinical features of phencyclidine (PCP) intoxication?

1. Neurologic: Vertical or horizontal <u>nystagmus,</u> numbness, <u>ataxia,</u> dysarthria, <u>muscle rigidity.</u>
2. Autonomic: <u>Hypertension,</u> <u>increased bronchial</u> and <u>salivary</u> <u>secretions.</u>
3. Mental: Hyperacusis, <u>labile</u> <u>affect,</u> agitation and assaultiveness.

PCP binds to N-methyl-D-aspartate (NMDA) subtype of glutamate receptors.

Intoxication with what substance has the cluster of symptoms of ataxia, nystagmus, muscular rigidity, normal or small pupils, and stupor?

PCP.

What is the medical complication commonly associated with PCP abuse?

Rhabdomyolysis.

According to the *Diagnostic and Statistical Manual of Mental Disorders, Fourth Revision* (DSM-IV), what are the differences between the diagnostic criteria for substance abuse and dependence?

In both diagnoses, the condition must have persisted for a 12-month period.

Abuse consists of any of the following: Continued substance use despite interpersonal problems; failure to fulfill obligations, physical hazards caused by substance use and recurrent substance-related legal problems; social/occupational dysfunction.

Dependence consists of three of the following: Tolerance, withdrawal, use of increasing amounts of a substance, <u>an unsuccessful attempt at cessation,</u> spending of considerable time in use of a substance, dysfunction, and continuing use despite problems.

When criteria for both abuse and dependence are met, the diagnosis is dependence.

What criteria differentiate substance dependence from substance abuse?

<u>Tolerance and withdrawal,</u> use of a substance in larger amounts and/or for longer periods than wanted, failure to reduce the use of a

substance, considerable time spent in substance use.

What are the symptoms of intoxication with *cannabis sativa*?

Conjunctival injection, increased appetite, dry mouth, and tachycardia with behavioral changes.

What is the average half-life of marijuana (tetrahydrocannabinol metabolites) in the human body?

From 2 to 7 weeks.

For what is the pentobarbital challenge test used?

Estimating the starting dose for barbiturate detoxification.

What psychopharmacologic agents are indicated to treat PCP intoxication?

Antipsychotic agents and benzodiazepines.

What are the clinical features of amphetamine abuse/dependence?

Chronic abuse of amphetamines may cause intracerebral vasculitis and hemorrhage.

Amphetamine withdrawal may cause vivid, unpleasant dreams.

Vivid, unpleasant dreams occur upon withdrawal from cocaine or amphetamine.

Cook and dream! (Coc-Am-Dream)

What are the risk factors for completed suicide in persons who have a chemical dependency problem?

DEAD:

D: Drug (history of drug overdose).

E: Ethanol (use of alcohol concurrently with drugs).

A: Abrupt (abrupt decision to commit suicide).

D: Desperate (recent interpersonal loss).

Withdrawal from what substance can cause insomnia, extreme anxiety and tremulousness, and grand mal seizure?

Sedating agents such as diazepam, alcohol, barbiturates.

Chapter 8 Psychotic Disorders, Mood Disorders, and Anxiety Disorders

What is dementia praecox?

The former name for schizophrenia.

Emil Kraepelin was the first author to describe the disease, calling it dementia praecox (literally "early-onset" dementia).

Eugen Bleuler renamed it as schizophrenia.

What was the important insight that made Emil Kraepelin an important figure in the history of psychiatry?

That major mental illnesses have different courses and outcomes.

Kraepelin believed that schizophrenia follows a course of declining cognition (hence the name "dementia praecox"), but that bipolar affective disorder does not.

What are common symptoms of water intoxication?

1. Tremor, ataxia, and restlessness.
2. Diarrhea and vomiting.
3. Polyuria.
4. Eventual stupor.

About 20% of patients with chronic schizophrenia drink water excessively, and 4% suffer from chronic hyponatremia and episodic water intoxication. However, the inappropriate secretion of antidiuretic hormone caused

*by antipsychotic agents,
carbamazepine, lithium, or other drugs
can cause the similar symptoms.*

What are the differences between paranoid and disorganized schizophrenia?

In paranoid schizophrenia the onset is late, thought processes are more linear, and the outcome is usually better.

In disorganized schizophrenia onset is early, thought processes are more disorganized, and the outcome is poor.

What types of hallucination may occur in association with the delusional theme in delusional disorder?

Tactile and olfactory hallucinations may occur in delusional disorder. Auditory or visual hallucinations are rare.

What are the negative symptoms in schizophrenia?

Flat affect, alogia (poverty of speech), and avolition.

What are the factors associated with a good prognosis in schizophrenia?

Before onset:

Good premorbid functioning, with little prodrome.

Onset:

Late age.

Acute onset of disease.

Symptoms:

Positive symptoms.

Confusion or perplexity at the height of the psychotic episode.

Other:

Female gender.

Absence of a family history of psychotic illness.

How to diagnose substance-induced mood disorder?

Mood symptoms must appear <u>after the onset of substance use.</u>

Mood symptoms may appear during intoxication or withdrawal. However, in order to make the diagnosis of substance-induced mood disorder instead of a diagnosis of substance intoxication or substance withdrawal, symptoms must <u>exceed those usually associated with intoxication or withdrawal,</u> and must be <u>severe enough to warrant clinical attention.</u>

What are the sleep abnormalities that may be detected with electroencephalogram (EEG) in patients with depression?

1. <u>Shortened latency of rapid-eye-movement (REM) sleep.</u>
2. Increased length of first REM episode.
3. Increased REM density.
4. <u>Decreased stage IV sleep.</u>
5. <u>Increased awakening during the second half of the night.</u>

Basic sleep-cycle EEG:

Awake: Fully awake (random fast waves); drowsiness (alpha waves).
Non-rapid-eye-movement (NREM) stage I (theta waves), stage II (theta waves with sleep spindles and K-complexes), stages III and IV (delta waves).
REM: Random fast waves with sawteeth.

What are the symptoms of major depressive disorder?

Major symptoms include: <u>Insomnia, weight loss, agitation, fatigue,</u> depressed mood, anhedonia, inappropriate feelings of guilt, difficulty in concentration, suicidal ideation/suicide attempt.

What are clinical features of post-traumatic stress disorder (PTSD)?

Exposure to a traumatic event and

<u>Re-experiencing of the event.</u>

<u>Increased arousal.</u>

<u>Avoidance of stimuli.</u>

Numbing of general responsiveness.

Persistence of symptoms for longer than 1 month.

What are the common sequelae experienced by persons who have been raped?

Feelings of shame, PTSD, and sexual difficulties.

What symptom is highly correlated with suicide in patients with schizophrenia?

Command hallucinations.

How is uncomplicated ("normal") bereavement differentiated from major depressive disorder?

After a beloved one's death, a patient with uncomplicated bereavement may:

Blame God, feel anger at God.

Have crying spells.

Feel extreme sadness.

Uncomplicated bereavement should NOT present with:

Suicidal ideation.

Guilt.

Psychomotor retardation.

Hallucination.

Preoccupation with worthlessness.

Symptoms lasting longer than 2 months.

Chapter 9 Somatoform Disorders, Eating Disorders, Sexuality Disorders, Sleep Disorders, Personality Disorders, and Culture-Bound Syndromes

What diagnoses are categorized as somatoform disorders?

The following seven diagnoses are offered in the *Diagnostic and Statistical Manual of the American Psychiatric Association, Fourth Revision* (DSM-IV) under the category of somatoform disorders:

1. Somatization disorder (also known as <u>Briquet's syndrome</u>).
2. <u>Conversion disorder.</u>
3. <u>Hypochondriasis.</u>
4. Pain disorder.
5. <u>Body dysmorphic disorder.</u>
6. Undifferentiated somatoform disorder.
7. Somatoform disorder not otherwise specified.

What is conversion disorder?

Conversion disorder consists of <u>neurologic</u> symptoms that cannot be explained by a known medical disorder. The symptoms are <u>not intentionally produced,</u> and <u>not limited to pain or sexual dysfunction.</u> Psychological factors are judged to be associated with the symptoms.

If non-neurologic symptoms are present, somatization disorder should be considered as a diagnosis.

If symptoms are intentionally produced, factitious disorder or malingering should be considered.

If only pain or sexual dysfunction is present, pain or sexual disorders should be considered.

What medical conditions have presentations similar to that of somatization disorder?

Many medical conditions have presentations similar to that of somatization disorder. Common ones include:

Multiple sclerosis.

Acute intermittent porphyria.

Systemic lupus erythematosus.

Fibromyositis.

Endocrine disorders.

Chronic infections.

What is the most common electrolyte imbalance seen in eating disorders?

Hypokalemia.

When cardiac disturbance (anxiety, palpitation) is suspected, check the patient's serum potassium concentration.

What are the major complications of anorexia nervosa?

General: <u>Cathexia, edema,</u> lanugo, electrolyte imbalance, decreased body temperature.

Mental: Depression.

Cardiac: <u>Loss of cardiac muscle,</u> change in heart rate.

Gastrointestinal: Digestive dysfunction.

Sexual: <u>Amenorrhea.</u>

Hematologic: Leukopenia.

Musculoskeletal: Osteoporosis, dental erosion.

What would the laboratory workup show in an adolescent girl with anorexia nervosa?

Low hematocrit, high cortisol, and high blood urea nitrogen concentration.

In comparison to patients with anorexia nervosa, what is characteristic in patients with involuntary starvation?

<u>A reduced activity level.</u>

Patients with eating disorders usually have an increased activity level.

What pharmacologic treatment is used for eating disorders?

Antidepressants with <u>serotonin-specific reuptake inhibitors (SSRIs)</u> the agents of first choice.

Tricyclic antidepressants such as imipramine and desipramine, as well as monoamine oxidase inhibitors, are helpful, but these are not the first choice if SSRIs were available.

Mirtazapine and venlafaxine are not well studied in eating disorders.

Bupropion is contraindicated in eating disorders.

A patient complains of snoring at night, and being irritable and drowsy during the daytime. What diagnostic test should be ordered?

Polysomnography.

What are the respiratory manifestations of sleep apnea?

Central: Lack of inspiratory effort.

Obstructive: Increased inspiratory effort.

What are clinical features of narcolepsy?

Episodes of sudden onset of sleep occurring daily for more than 3 months, and which present with one or both of the following features:

1. Cataplexy (sudden loss of muscle tone, often precipitated by strong emotion), followed by the patient's entry into rapid-

eye-movement (REM) sleep
within a few minutes after
falling asleep;

2. Repeated intrusions of REM
sleep into the transition
between sleep and wakefulness
(as manifested by hypnopompic
or hypnagogic hallucinations or
sleep paralysis).

What is the first choice in initial treatment for primary insomnia?

Sleep hygiene (restricting the use of the bed to sleep only).

What observations are characteristic during REM sleep?

Tachycardia.

Penile tumescence.

Atonia.

Rapid eye movements.

Dreaming.

Relatively low-voltage mixed-frequency waves in the electroencephalogram.

What characteristics are usually reported of patients with obstructive sleep apnea?

Obesity.

Frequent daytime napping.

Snoring at bedtime.

Early-morning awakening and inability to return to sleep are associated with what clinical conditions?

Depression.

Advanced sleep-phase syndrome.

Alcohol abuse.

Mania.

What is the most appropriate initial intervention for sleep apnea?

Continuous positive airway pressure (CPAP).

What are typical presentations of narcissistic personality disorder?

Arrogance.

Haughty behavior.

Belief by the subject that he or she is special.

Need for excessive admiration.

Envy of others.

Lack of empathy.

Sense of entitlement.

Interpersonal exploitativeness.

Grandiosity; extreme sense of self-importance.

What clinical features might differentiate borderline personality disorder from histrionic personality disorder?

Both disorders are marked by labile affect, seductiveness, exaggerated anger, and volatile relationships.

Self-mutilation is frequent in patients with borderline personality disorder.

What is sleep terror syndrome?

A subtype of parasomnia.

It is characterized by recurrent episodes of abrupt awakening from sleep, usually during the first third of a major sleep episode, with a panicky scream, intensive fear, and signs of autonomic arousal during each episode.

The patient is usually relatively unresponsive to the efforts of others to comfort him or her.

No detailed dream is recalled.

Sleep terror syndrome is more frequent in children than in adults.

In nightmare disorder, the details of dreams can be recalled. Awakening in this disorder usually occurs in the second half of the sleep period.

What are the most and least prevalent male sexuality disorders?

Most prevalent: Male erectile disorder.

Least prevalent: Male orgasmic disorder.

What is fetishism?

A condition in which an individual is sexually aroused by nonliving objects, such as undergarments or high-heeled shoes. Male persons with this disorder may be caught <u>stealing women's clothing.</u>

What is the main symptom of transvestic fetishism?

Cross-dressing.

Which sexual and gender identity disorder primarily involves <u>homosexual individuals?</u>

None. According to the American Psychiatric Association, homosexuality is a life style rather than a pathologic phenomenon.

What is homophobia?

A persistently negative attitude toward or fear of homosexuality or homosexuals.

What is dyspareunia?

Recurrent or persistent genital pain associated with sexual intercourse. It may occur in either male or female individuals, and can happen before or after intercourse. Both medical and psychological conditions can contribute to its development.

What is the minimum time criterion for the diagnosis of paraphilia?

Six months.

What does the nocturnal penile tumescence monitoring test evaluate?

Erectile capacity.

What is *attaque de nervios*?	A culture-restricted syndrome among <u>Latino persons from the Caribbean.</u> It is marked by shouting, crying, trembling, anger, a sensation of heat in the chest and head, headache, verbal and physical aggression, insomnia, and despair. It includes no acute fear (as distinguished from panic attack). Persons with attaque de nervios may experience amnesia, but rapidly return to their usual functional state.
What is Couvade syndrome?	A culture-bound syndrome in which a father takes his bed during or shortly after the birth of his child, as though he himself had given birth.
What is Amok?	A culture-bound syndrome found in <u>Malayans.</u> It appears as a dissociative episode with a violent outburst. Accompanying symptoms include persecutory delusions, automatism, and <u>amnesia.</u>

Chapter 10 Forensic Psychiatry

What was the legal principle formulated after the case of Tarasoff versus The Board of Regents of the University of California?

The clinician has the responsibility to warn the intended victims of dangerous patients, and to take steps to protect the intended victims.

What is paternalism?

A physician acting in the best interest of a patient whose own capability of autonomous decision making is severely impaired.

What is the commonly quoted code of ethics of the American Psychiatric Association?

It is a psychiatrist's obligation to report other psychiatrists' unethical behavior.

It is unethical to accept a commission for patient referrals.

It is unethical to have sexual relationships with patients.

It is unethical to participate in a legally authorized execution.

What are the requirements of the Patient Self-Determination Act for patients admitted to a hospital?

Patients must receive written or printed information advising them of their right to refuse treatment, to ask for advance directives, and to designate a health-care proxy.

What is required by the concept of informed consent?

Informed consent requires a thorough discussion with the patient of the:

1. The indications for treatment.
2. Risks from treatment.
3. Adverse effects of treatment.
4. Alternative forms of treatment.
5. Risks of not having treatment.

To be able to give informed consent, a patient must have <u>sufficient information</u> to understand the treatment and to be <u>mentally competent</u> to make a <u>voluntary choice</u> about having or not having it.

What should a psychiatrist find when evaluating a patient's competency to make a will?

The patient should know that:

1. He or she is making a will.
2. How the will distributes his or her property.
3. The nature and extent of his or her property subject to distribution by the will.
4. The persons who would normally be expected to benefit from the will.

If a psychiatrist who is a former employee of an institution wants to write articles for publication about his or her clinical cases while at the institution, what steps should the psychiatrist take?

The psychiatrist should keep a separate set of process notes, which are <u>his or her personal property rather than the property of the institution.</u>

According to the American Psychiatric Association and the World Psychiatric Association, can a psychiatrist participate in the legal execution of a prisoner by administering a lethal dose of a sedative/hypnotic drug?

No. Both organizations consider this behavior to be <u>unethical, and maintain that psychiatrists should not participate in executions.</u>

What is the legal principle most relevant to the administration of medications?

Informed consent.

What should a patient be told when undergoing a psychiatric examination to determine suitability for a job?

That the examination is <u>not confidential,</u> and that there is <u>no therapeutic alliance</u> with the psychiatrist giving the examination.

What ethical principle provides the most appropriate basis for psychiatric intervention in the case of a mentally incompetent patient?

Beneficence.

What is the usual basis for most psychiatrists to prescribe a medication that is not approved by the FDA?

That the medication is <u>probably effective for the patient's problem, on the basis of available data.</u>

What is fiduciary duty?

The responsibility of a physician to act in a patient's best interests.

What is the term used for a patient's legal right to bar his or her physician from revealing treatment matters in court?

Privilege.

What are the indications for seclusion and restraint of a patient?

1. Prevention of harm to the patient or others.
2. Use of seclusion and restraint as ongoing behavioral treatments and to decrease stimulation.
3. <u>Non-use of seclusion and restraint as a punishment</u> for violence.

What is the most important factor in determining the competency of a patient who refuses a recommended therapeutic procedure?

The patient's understanding of the medical consequences of not undergoing the procedure.

Chapter 11 Consultation-Liaison Psychiatry

What is the mechanism of menopause?

It is the progressive insensitivity of the ovary to the effect of follicle-stimulating hormone (FSH).

What conditions may cause catatonia?

Conditions that may cause catatonia are:

Mania.

Neurologic disorders (e.g., encephalitis).

Depression.

Schizophrenia.

Ingestion of phencyclidine.

Other psychiatric conditions.

Electrolyte imbalances, such as hypocalcemia, do not cause catatonia.

What is the drug of choice for rapid tranquilization?

Haloperidol given intramuscularly.

If the patient is willing and able to take an oral drug, the choice would be equivocal. Recent research shows risperidone to be as effective as haloperidol and to have a comparably rapid onset of action and a better side-

effect profile. This use of risperidone, however, has not yet become a standard practice.

What is the major concern in acetaminophen overdose?

Hepatotoxicity.

What are some important factors in evaluating chronic pain?

The patient's <u>ethnic background</u> may influence the symptoms.

<u>Depression</u> may present as chronic pain.

One third of patients respond to a <u>placebo.</u>

What medical conditions should be ruled out in patients with acute extreme anxiety?

<u>Alcohol withdrawal.</u>

<u>Pulmonary embolism.</u>

Use of sympathomimetic agents.

What is the most useful diagnostic procedure for patients with suspected delirium?

The Mini-Mental Status Examination (MMSE).

What is the role of benzodiazepines in controlling delirium?

As a general rule, benzodiazepines should be avoided in cases of delirium. Benzodiazepines may cause increased confusion, disinhibition, falling, and behavioral problems.

What is the best agent for managing steroid-induced mania?

Usually, a low dose antipsychotic agent, because of these drugs' rapid effect.

Benzodiazepines may cause more confusion.

Antidepressants and mood-stabilizing drugs take weeks to produce effects, and are therefore not used.

What characteristics are more likely in elderly than in young patients with medical surgical conditions?

Delirium.

Adverse reactions to anticholinergic drugs.

What is the most important risk factor for postpartum psychosis?

A history of puerperal psychiatric illness.

Age, complications of delivery, and multiparity are not risk factors for postpartum psychosis.

What are the essential responsibilities for a physician requesting a psychiatric consultation?

The physician should prepare the patient for the consultation and clearly state the reason for, urgency of, and expectations from the consultation.

What symptoms may acute intermittent porphyria present, and what test could be diagnostic for this condition?

The symptoms of acute intermittent porphyria include colicky abdominal pain with nausea and vomiting, psychosis (e.g., hallucinations), agitated depression, and polyneuropathy.

Acute intermittent porphyria has been estimated to be undiagnosed in 0.5% of psychiatric patients.

The clinical diagnostic test for the condition is the <u>porphobilinogen</u> test.

If a postsurgical patient reports inadequate pain relief after having intramuscular (IM) meperidine formula replaced by oral (PO) meperidine at the same dosage and frequency, what is likely to be the reason for this problem?

Meperidine PO has a lower analgesic potency than IM meperidine.

What is the earliest symptom of delirium?

<u>Impaired attention.</u> Mood fluctuation, agitation, insomnia, and psychosis may follow.

What is the neuropsychiatric presentation of human immunodeficiency virus infection?

<u>Memory impairment (dementia).</u>

<u>Pathologic slowing of information processing.</u>

<u>Dysgraphia</u>

<u>Leg weakness.</u>

Delirium.

Anxiety disorders.

Adjustment disorders.

Depressive disorders.

Substance abuse.

What should be done for a terminally ill patient who is in the bargaining stage of reacting to his or her impending death?

Assure the patient he or she will be given the best care regardless of the patient's behavior.

What should be done for a patient who is in denial of an untreatable illness?

Ensure that the patient has been informed about the illness and the treatment that can be given for it.

What is the most important principle in helping dying patients?

Preserve the patient's hope.

What is malingering?

The <u>intentional</u> production of false or grossly exaggerated physical or psychological symptoms, <u>motivated by external incentives.</u>

What psychiatric symptoms might be related to left-frontal-lobe damage?

Depression.

How do questions about suicide influence patients' suicidal behavior?

Questions about suicide do not influence the likelihood of a suicide attempt.

What is the most common mental disorder of elderly patients with acute and chronic medical conditions in primary-care settings?	Depression.
What is neurasthenia?	A term used to describe the condition currently considered as chronic fatigue syndrome. *Neurasthenia is still a popular diagnosis in China.*
In what malignant condition can the initial presentation be depression?	Carcinoma of the pancreas.
What agents may be used to prevent akathisia (anxiety, agitation, fidgeting, need to move constantly, and a strong sensation of being uncomfortable)?	Beta-blockers (treatment of choice). <u>Benzodiazepines.</u> Anticholinergic agents. Amantadine. Clonidine.

A patient had a head concussion 4 days before being brought to psychiatric attention. He was doing well until 2 hours ago, when his mental status began to change. What is the test of choice?

Magnetic resonance imaging is preferred to computed tomography. An imaging scan should be done before a spinal tap. Radiography of the skull or electroencephalography is not diagnostic.

What is the best psychiatric group-treatment strategy for patients with metastasized breast cancer?

Supportive expressive group therapy.

What is the best group-treatment strategy for patients at risk for acquired immune deficiency syndrome (AIDS)?

Educational groups.

What psychiatric medication may exacerbate symptoms of psoriasis?

Lithium.

What medication is indicated for severe alcohol withdrawal?

A benzodiazepine.

How do antidepressants influence the seizure threshold?

Serotonin-specific reuptake inhibitors may not influence the seizure threshold.

Bupropion, tricyclic antidepressants, and tetracyclic antidepressants may lower seizure threshold.

With what neuropsychiatric symptoms can digitalis toxicity present?

Depression.

Manic-like behavior.

Agitation.

Visual abnormalities with scotoma, flickering halos, and objects appearing to have yellow-green borders.

What are typical symptoms of vitamin B$_{12}$ deficiency?

Abnormal proprioception.

Dysethesia.

Dementia.

Macrocytic anemia.

When a patient in a medical unit develops dysarthria with a protruding tongue and torticollis, what medication should be suspected?

An antiemetic such as:

Metoclopramide (Reglan).

Promethazine (Phenergan).

Prochlorperazine (Compazine).

These medications are widely used in medical units. They have dopamine-antagonistic effects and may cause extrapyramidal side-effects.

What is catatonia and how is it treated?

Catatonia is a cluster of symptoms that may present with:

Motoric immobility (catalepsy or stupor).

Excessive motor activity.

Extreme negativism (rigid posture upon externally attempted movements).

Mutism.

Peculiarities of voluntary movement (bizarre postures).

Stereotyped movements.

Prominent mannerisms.

Prominent grimacing.

Echolalia.

Echopraxia.

The treatment of choice is a benzodiazepine. Lorazepam given intramuscularly has well-documented efficacy in catatonia.

Catatonia occurs most commonly in bipolar affective disorder (45% of cases) and neurologic disease (40% of cases), and much less often in schizophrenia (5% to 10% of cases).

What is postconcussional disorder?

After a head-trauma accident that causes significant cerebral concussion, the affected individual may display:

Difficulty in focusing attention or with memory.

Headache.

Vertigo or dizziness.

Irritability.

Emotional lability.

Depression.

Fatigue.

Disturbed sleep.

Changes in personality.

Apathy or lack of spontaneity.

These symptoms should last at least 3 months for a diagnosis of postconcussional disorder.

Chapter 12 Child Psychiatry

When does gender identity become fixed?

At the age of 2 to 3 years.

What factors must be ruled out in the diagnosis of enuresis?

Organic factors, such as urinary tract infections. Urinalysis is usually ordered, but more sophisticated studies should be deferred until proven to be necessary.

What medical conditions should be ruled out before making a diagnosis of encopresis?

Hirschsprung's disease and other conditions that may cause fecal retention. Physical examination, abdominal radiography, and fecal examination may be indicated.

What psychiatric symptom is highly associated with Tourette's syndrome?

Obsessions and compulsions.

What pharmacologic treatments are used for Tourette's syndrome?

Haloperidol.

Pimozide.

Clonidine.

At what age do children with Tourette's syndrome start to present with symptoms?

Between 6 and 10 years of age.

What is the stage at which a child with a congenital physical deformity is most vulnerable to emotional disturbance?	Early adolescence (age 11 to 15 years).
At what age does a child begin to preferentially look and listen to his mother?	One week.
What is a transitional object?	An infant's "not-me" possession, usually a reassuring blanket or toy, that preserves the illusion of the comforting maternal object even in her absence. *The concept of transitional object was coined by Donald W. Winnicot.*
What are the basics of Heinz Kohut's theory of personality?	Individuals (selves) need <u>empathic interaction</u> with their mother and other family members (objects). This interaction is called <u>self-object function.</u> Failure of self-object function may lead to developmental arrest and personality disorders.
What is egocentrism?	A characteristic feature of children in the preoperational stage (2 to 7 years). Children in this stage see themselves as the center of the universe. They are unable to take the

role of another person. For example, a child may hold a picture facing toward himself, and ask his mother about images in the picture, not realizing that his mother can only see the back of the picture.

Jean Piaget's developmental stages are the:

Sensorimotor (0 to 2 years).
Preoperational (2 to 7 years).
Concrete operational (7 to 11 years).
Formal operational (11 years onward).

At what age does stranger anxiety develop?

Stranger anxiety is first noted at the age of 7 months, and develops fully at the age of 8 months.

What is the psychoanalytic explanation for the trends in adolescents' unreasoning passion toward celebrity stars and cult figures?

In psychoanalytic theory, it is believed that this phenomenon is related to the direction of adolescents' feelings away from parents and their unconscious displacement of incestuous thoughts.

What are the cognitive developmental characteristics in the formal operational stage of Jean Piaget's theory of development?

Beyond 12 years of age, an individual is able to deal with concepts and ideas. This pattern of thinking and reasoning is described as abstract, deductive, and conceptual.

Synthesis, the integration of traits, attitudes, and impulses to create a total personality, is an important task in this stage.

Characteristics of Piaget's other developmental stages are as follows:

Sensorimotor stage: Stereotyped reaction to stimuli; object permanency develops during the second year of life.

Preoperational stage: Symbolic functions develop; egocentric thinking magical thinking; basic moral thought occurs (good versus bad).

Concrete operational stage: Rational and logical thought; the concept of conservation (water in a tall cup has the same volume as in a bowl); ability to understand someone else's point of view.

What is infantile amnesia?

Most people cannot recall events that happened before 5 years of age. This phenomenon is called "infantile amnesia." It is probably caused by the lack of language-based retrieval of prelinguistic memory.

According to whose theory, is <u>good-enough mothering</u> important in providing a suppportive environment to infants?

Good-enough mothering is an essential concept in Donald W. Winnicott's object-relation theory.

Another important concept of Winnicott is that of the transitional object.

What is the theory of <u>separation–individuation?</u>

The separation–individuation theory, proposed by <u>Margaret Mahler,</u> describes how young children acquire a sense of identity apart from mothers.

Rapprochement is the most frequently mentioned stage of Mahler's theory. This French word means "reconciliation." In the stage of rapprochement, children constantly are concerned about the actual physical location of their mothers, and have great need for maternal love. Lack of maternal love or absence of the mother during the rapprochement stage may lead to a child's anger (<u>temper tantrums, whining behavior, moodiness</u>) and has been linked to the pathogenesis of borderline personality disorder.

According to Mahler's theory, the six stages of separation-individuation are:

1. *Normal autism (birth to 2 months).*
2. *Symbiosis (2 to 5 months).*
3. *Differentiation (5 to 10 months).*

4. Practicing (10 to 18 months).
5. Rapprochement (18 to 24 months).
6. Object constancy (2 to 5 years).

What are the characteristics of Asperger's disorder? How can Asperger's disorder be differentiated from autistic disorder (Kanner's autism)?

Asperger's disorder is a disorder within the spectrum of autism. It is characterized by:

1. Poor social interaction (deficiencies in <u>eye gaze,</u> facial expression, body language, <u>poor peer relationships, and lack of social reciprocity and interests</u>).
2. A stereotyped or repetitive pattern of behavior.
3. Usually normal <u>language</u> development and <u>intelligence quotient (IQ).</u>

<u>Autistic disorder,</u> also known as Kanner's autism, has the same symptoms as Asperger's disorder, but is further marked by <u>poor development in language and/or symbolic/imaginative play,</u> and an IQ below 70 in 70% of cases.

What is the most important domain in finding abnormalities for a diagnosis of autistic disorder?

<u>Interpersonal relations</u>/social interaction.

Other important domains in which abnormalities characteristic of autism may be found are communications and stereotyped patterns of behavior, interest, and activities.

What is the most important prognostic factor related to long-term outcome in infantile autism?

Language development.

What are the adverse effects of methylphenidate (Ritalin)?

Emotional lability, weight loss, insomnia, decreasing TCA concentration, and rebound hyperactivity.

What are the choices of pharmacologic treatment for attention-deficit/hyperactivity disorder (AD/HD)?

Stimulants: Methylphenidate (Ritalin) is usually the agent of first - choice. Dextroamphetamine (Dexedrine) and amphetamine (Adderall) may be used as first-choice or alternative agents. Pemoline (Cylert) may cause liver failure. (Note: Discontinuation of a stimulant may induce rebound symptoms such as hyperactivity, irritability, excitability, and talkativeness.)

Antidepressants: Bupropion (Wellbutrin) and other antidepressants.

Clonidine.

What are the differences in the diagnostic criteria for a major depressive episode in children as compared to adults?

In children, the diagnostic criteria for a major depressive episode are the same as for adults, except that:

1. Mood change can present as irritable mood instead of

depressed mood, and prepubertal children have <u>more frequent episodes of irritable mood</u> than do adult depressive patients.
2. Instead of significant weight loss, children with depression may present failure to make expected weight gains.

What are the manifestations of major depressive disorder in children?

Children with major depression may be <u>irritable,</u> and their school grades may decline, but they should have a <u>good previous level of functioning.</u> Hallucination can occur. It is also very important to recognize that unexplained <u>somatic symptoms</u> are often a clue to depression.

What is the most common emergency diagnosis in child and adolescent psychiatry?

Threat of suicide.

What characteristic of manic disorder is more likely in prepubertal children than in adult patients?

Irritability as opposed to euphoria.

At what age do children start to understand that death is permanent?

Seven years.

What is the most effective treatment for conduct disorder?

Behavior therapy. An effective behavior therapy plan for conduct disorder should include environmental structure and <u>parent management training.</u>

What is introjection?

Internalizing the qualities of an object, as in the case of a child who mentally incorporates a model of his mother as a soothing presence.

Projection (narcissistic defense) consists of perceiving and reacting to unacceptable inner impulses and their derivatives as though they were outside the self.

Identification is an unconscious defense mechanism in which the characteristics and qualities of another person or object are incorporated into the subject's ego system.

When does the synaptogenesis of neural circuitry in brain development reach its peak?

At the toddler stage (2 to 3 years).

Which type of memory do the hippocampus and parahippocampal gyrus mediate?

Declarative memory.

Though the concept is controversial, memory is tentatively classified as nondeclarative and declarative. Nondeclarative memory (also known as "implicit memory") cannot be expressed in words. It does not require focal, conscious attention. It usually remains intact after brain injury.

Nondeclarative memory deals with skills (procedural), habits, priming (see below), simple classical conditioning, and nonassociative learning.

Probable brain structures involved in nondeclarative memory include the basal ganglia, limbic system (amygdala, anterior cingulate gyrus, orbitofrontal cortex), and perceptual cortices.

Declarative memory (also known as "explicit memory") requires conscious awareness and concentration. It is this type of memory that is mainly impaired after brain injury.

Declarative memory deals with facts and events.

Probable structures involved in declarative memory include the hippocampus, orbitofrontal cortex (overlapping with nondeclarative memory), and parahippocampal gyrus.

Priming is facilitation of the ability to identify stimuli on the basis of recent experience with the same stimuli. For example, amnestic patients may show a normal tendency to complete three-letter stems on the basis of previously encountered words.

What type of memory is skill and habits?

Implicit memory (nondeclarative type).

What type of memory is used in storing autobiographical information?

Explicit memory (declarative type).

What are the first signs of onset of puberty in girls?

Pubic hair growth and breast enlargement.

Stages of puberty in girls:

1. *No pubic hair; elevation of papillae alone.*
2. *Sparse growth of yellowish hair along the labia. Budding of breasts.*
3. *Pubic hair becomes darker, coarser, and more curled, but is still sparse. Breasts become enlarged and elevated.*
4. *Adult-type pubic hair begins growing, but the area covered is small, and there is no coverage to the medial thighs. Breasts become more enlarged.*
5. *Adult distribution of pubic hair. Mature breasts.*

Stages of puberty in boys:

1. *No pubic hair. Testes, scrotum, and penis are the same as in early childhood.*
2. *Sparse growth of yellowish hair at the base of the penis. Scrotum and testes are slightly enlarged. Scrotal skin is reddened. No enlargement of penis.*
3. *Pubic hair becomes darker, coarser, and more curled, but is still sparse. Penis is slightly enlarged, mainly in length.*
4. *Adult-type pubic hair, but the area covered is small, with no coverage to the medial thighs. Penis is further enlarged, with growth in breadth. Development of glans. Testes and scrotum are larger. Scrotal skin is darker.*
5. *Adult distribution of pubic hair. Mature genitals.*

What is the first physical change during female sexual development?

A growth spurt in height.

At what psychoanalytic stage do children learn to manage triangular relationships?

The Oedipal stage.

The developmental stages according to Sigmund Freud were the:

Oral stage (0 to 1 year): Focusing on feeding.

Anal stage (1 to 3 years): Focusing on bowel functioning.

Phallic stage (3 to 5 years): Focusing on the genitalia, and including:

The Oedipal complex, in which the child falls in love with the parent of the opposite sex and tries to eliminate the other parent.
Castration anxiety, in which a boy fears that his father will cut off his penis.
Penis envy, in which a girl wishes to have a penis.

Latency (6 to 11 years), in which sexual development is stagnant.

Adolescence (12 to 18 years).

What are the major fears of a 2½-year-old child who is hospitalized?

Separation and abandonment.

At what age does stranger anxiety occur?

Eight to 10 months.

At what age does a child first recognize its mother's face?

Two to 3 months.

Social developmental milestones in childhood are:

Six weeks: Social smile.

Two to 3 months: Recognition of mother.

Eight to 10 months: Stranger anxiety and playing peek-a-boo.

Twelve months: Drinking from a cup.

Fourteen to 18 months: Imitating housework.

Twenty-four months: Playing interactive games.

Four years: Dressing self with supervision.

Five years: Dressing alone.

Which defense mechanism best characterizes the behavior of an adolescent girl who cleans her room meticulously after a heated argument with her mother about her miniskirt?

Sublimation.

Displacement (neurotic defenses): Shifting an emotion or drive cathexis from one idea or object to another that resembles the original idea or object in some aspect or quality.

Repression (neurotic defenses): Expelling or withholding from consciousness an idea or feeling.

Children with Turner's syndrome are most likely to manifest what sexual behavior during adulthood?

Heterosexuality.

In what was Jean Piaget most interested?

The processes that children use to arrive at answers.

What persons are legally required to report child abuse?

Teachers, physicians, district attorneys, and hospital activity therapists.

In the emergency room of a hospital, a young child holds his familiar blanket. As what does this blanket serve?

A transitional object.

A 2-year-old child knows to look for a toy hidden under a blanket. What is this phenomenon called?

Object permanence.

In his cognitive development theory, Jean Piaget describes four stages:

Sensorimotor stage (0 to 18 to approximately 24 months): Object permanency develops.
Preoperational thought–prelogical (2 to 6 years): Symbolic functions develop. Egocentric thinking (everything revolves around the child) and magical thinking occur.
Concrete operations (7 to 11 years): Concept of conservation of volume (beaker-of-water experiment) occurs.
Formal operations (12+ years): Abstract thinking, deductive reasoning, and conceptual thinking develop.

What is concrete operation?

At the age of 7 to 11 years, children start having rational and logical thought processes, and apply a more conceptual framework to the world. However, they still lack abstract thinking, deductive reasoning, and conceptual thinking abilities.

At what stage of Erik Erikson's life-cycle theory is a child who strives to achieve a sense of self-control and free will, struggling between cooperation and willfulness?

Autonomy versus shame and doubt.

Erikson's epigenetic model of developmental stages posits the following stages:

Basic trust versus mistrust (0 to 1 year).

Autonomy versus shame and doubt (1 to 3 years).

Initiative versus guilt (3 to 6 years).

Industry versus inferiority (6 to 12 years).

Identity versus role confusion (12 to 20 years).

Intimacy versus isolation (20 to 40 years).

Generativity versus stagnation (40 to 65 years).

Ego integrity versus despair (65 years and beyond).

According to Erik Erikson, the developmental crisis most typical of normal middle age involves what?

Generativity.

A 4-year-old child's mother is out of town, but the child can reassure himself that his mother loves him even when she is away. What is this phenomenon called in Mahler's theory?

Object constancy.

The stages of Margaret Mahler's separation–individuation process are:

Symbiosis (0 to 5 months): The infant does not differentiate from the mother.

Differentiation (5 to 10 months): Physical movement away from the mother, and development of stranger anxiety.

Practicing (10 to 15 months): Great exploration and separation anxiety occur.

Rapprochement (18 to 24 months): Increased self-awareness makes child want to stay close to the mother, but the child also wants to explore.

Consolidation and object constancy (24 to 36 months): The child maintains an internal representation of the mother and tolerates separations.

What is the typical thought process during the preschool period?

Magical thinking.

When is cooperative play most likely to be seen?

From 32 to 60 months.

What diagnosis comorbid with AD/HD carries the worst prognosis?

Conduct disorder.

What are the efficacies of different modalities in treating obsessive compulsive disorder?

Serotonin-specific reuptake inhibitors and cognitive behavioral therapy are both effective.

What affects a child's psychological adjustment to the divorce of its parents?

The amount of parental conflict after the divorce.

What are the core features of Prader–Willi syndrome?

Mental retardation, obesity, short stature, hypogonadism, and hyperphagia. Chromosome 15 deletion exists in 70% of cases.

What is the core feature of Fragile X syndrome?

The triad of a long face, prominent ears, and macro-orchidism, with 80% of patients also having AD/HD.

The pathophysiology of Fragile X syndrome involves inactivation of the FMR-1 gene at Xq27.3, caused by multiple abnormal CGG base repeats.

What is the appropriate reaction to the parents of a 3-year-old child who has not begun to speak intelligibly?

Expression of some concern, because most children in this age can effectively make themselves understood. Appropriate evaluation may be suggested.

When young children need to be examined in the emergency-room setting, should their parents be allowed to stay with them?

Yes, so as to minimize the psychological trauma to the patients.

What behavior differentiates conduct disorder from other behavior disorders in a prepubertal child?

<u>Initiating fights,</u> bullying, <u>threatening or intimidation of others,</u> physical cruelty to people and/or animals, stealing, forcing of sex, arson and/or destruction of others' property, breaking into others' houses or automobiles, lying, staying out at night before the age of 13 years, running away from home, <u>truancy from school.</u>

What is the core feature of oppositional-defiant disorder?

The child does not respect authority figures, has a short temper, and easily becomes angry and resentful.

What is the first step in evaluating a 2-year-old child who does not speak?

Check audiometry.

What is the main clinical presentation of children with pediatric autoimmune neuropsychiatric disorders associated with streptococcal infection (PANDAS)?

Choreiform movements and obsessive–compulsive symptoms.

What are the characteristic features of Rett's disorder?

Normal prenatal, perinatal, and psychomotor development through the first 5 months after birth, and a normal head circumference at birth followed by:

- Deceleration of head growth beginning in early childhood (between the ages of 5 and 48 months).
- Loss of previously acquired purposeful hand skills and subsequent development of stereotyped hand movements (e.g., hand-wringing or handwashing).
- Loss of social engagement.
- Poor coordination in gait or trunk movement.
- Severe impairment of expressive and receptive language development, with severe psychomotor retardation.

What is most likely to be a manifestation of selective mutism in children?

Anxiety disorder.

What is frequently seen in the members of an incestuous family?

Denial of sexual content of behavior.

What is anaclitic depression?

Described by René Spitz, anaclitic depression refers to children who become depressed and nonresponsive after prolonged separation from their mothers.

How should one manage the school phobia associated with nonpsychotic separation anxiety in a preadolescent child?

Rapidly return the child to school.

Chapter 13 Psychosocial Therapies

What is the fundamental rule for psychoanalysis?

Free association.

What is working through?

A procedure in psychodynamic psychotherapy. Through the analyst's interpretation of transference and resistance, insight may finally become integrated into the patient's conscious awareness.

Besides being a conjunctive biologic treatment, does medication play a role in psychotherapy?

Medication prescribed by a psychiatrist may function as a psychological connection to the psychiatrist during the periods between visits.

What is the focus in interpersonal psychotherapy?

Patterns of communication.

For which patients is brief focal psychodynamic psychotherapy appropriate and for which patients is it contraindicated?

Patients suitable for brief focal psychodynamic psychotherapy must be highly motivated, able to deal with psychological concepts, and able to develop a therapeutic alliance.

Contraindications to such therapy are past suicide attempts, substance dependence, chronic alcohol abuse, incapacitating obsessional or phobic symptoms, and destructive behavior.

Brief focal psychodynamic psychotherapy was developed at the Tavistock Clinic in London by Daniel Malan.

Why is group therapy often an appropriate therapy for adolescents?

Adolescents are more comfortable with peers, especially when they have to hear and consider critical comments. They also tend to dislike authority such as that of the therapist, which is diminished in group sessions.

What should a therapist do if a patient begins acting seductively and requests closer contact, such as an evening appointment or dinner?

The therapist should first examine his or her own behavior and possible countertransference. Second, if appropriate, the therapist should discuss his or her observation with the patient and explore the meaning of the patient's behavior.

What conditions are considered appropriate for biofeedback therapy?

Neuromuscular conditions including pain, tension headaches, migraine headaches, neuromuscular rehabilitation, and seizure.

Cardiovascular conditions including hypertension, hypotension, cardiac arrhythmias, Raynaud's syndrome.

Gastrointestinal and genitourinary conditions including fecal incontinence and enuresis.

Pulmonary disease, consisting of asthma.

According to psychoanalytic theory, what is the etiology of the formation of a neurotic symptom?

Impaired ego function.

Failure of repression.

What factor correlates most strongly with a positive outcome of psychotherapy?

The therapist's <u>empathy.</u>

What is the essential technical goal of cognitive therapy?

Eliciting and testing <u>automatic thoughts.</u>

What is the therapeutic focus in supportive psychotherapy?

"Here and now"—coping with daily stresses.

What is double binding?

This concept, generated by Gregory Bateson, is used to describe a hypothetical family in which <u>children receive conflicting parental messages about their behavior, attitudes, and feelings.</u>

What are the five stages of reaction to approaching death developed by Elizabeth Kubler-Ross?

1. Shock and denial.
2. Anger.
3. Bargaining.
4. Depression.
5. Acceptance.

Treatment for a patient facing death is to recognize the reaction process and provide compassionate care.

What intervention techniques are utilized in a family-system approach to family therapy?

1. Giving the entire family specific homework assignments on which to work outside of treatment sessions.
2. Exploring the family's beliefs about the meaning of its members' behaviors.
3. Identifying family members' "problematic" behaviors and reframing them positively.
4. Directing members to engage in new behaviors during treatment sessions (e.g., changing seats), and observing the effects of this on patterns of behavior.

Family therapy should not identify the most dysfunctional family dyad and explicit work on that relationship initially.

What is the primary focus of behavior therapy in the treatment of anorexia nervosa?

Restoring proper body weight.

What does the conceptual model of the "triangle of insight" involve?

Transference patterns, current relationships, and past relationships.

According to Daniel Malan, interpretation of the triangle of insight is the ideal goal in brief psychodynamic psychotherapy.

What should the psychiatrist do when 10 minutes late for an appointment with a psychodynamic psychotherapy patient?

Apologize and arrange to make up the time.

What is the most common theme discussed in psychotherapy with elderly patients?

Loss.

What is an example of countertransference?

A psychiatrist's not wanting to work with alcoholic patients, and believing that they are "hopeless" and "completely unmotivated."

When is it optimal to use psychopharmacologic medications in connection with psychodynamic psychotherapy?

When the meanings and effects of medications as well as their connecting function between therapist and the patient are integrated into the patient's understanding.

What type of psychotherapy should be more applicable to patients who have repeated "nervous breakdowns" under stress?

Supportive rather than insight-orientated psychotherapy.

What are the indications for a supportive emphasis in psychotherapy?

Poor frustration tolerance and severely impaired object relations.

What is confrontation?

It addresses an issue that the patient does not want to accept, or identifies the patient's avoidance or minimization of an issue. Although often gentle, as practiced in psychotherapy, the concept of confrontation carries the unfortunate connotation in common parlance of aggressiveness or bluntness.

What is resistance?

Unconscious ideas or impulses that are repressed and prevented from reaching awareness because for some reason they are unacceptable to the patient's consciousness.

What are the indications for termination in psychodynamic psychotherapy?

The superego has been modified, the presenting symptoms have been eliminated, the patient's interpersonal relationships have improved, and the patient is independently able to recognize and examine conflicts.

A separated couple is in marital therapy with a psychodynamically oriented therapist. How should the therapist demonstrate therapeutic neutrality in this case?

The concept of therapeutic neutrality is demonstrated by inquiring about why the couple is considering divorce, and also why they are considering returning to their marriage, if this is the case.

What is the indication for dialectical behavior therapy?

Borderline personality disorder.

Dialectical behavior therapy was developed by Marsha Linehan.

What is "reframing" in family therapy?

Also called "positive connotation," reframing is a relabeling of all negatively expressed feelings or behaviors as positive.

What psychotherapeutic technique is most important in the treatment of patients who are suicidal?

Establishing a therapeutic alliance.

Chapter 14 Psychopharmacology and Other Biologic Therapies

Which antidepressants cause no sexual dysfunction?

<u>Bupropion,</u> mirtazapine and nefazodone.

What is the safety of antidepressants in pregnancy?

Because of the lack of convincing prospective data, this is not a fair question. Of note is that Class B antidepressants have been found safe in animal studies, Class C have shown adverse effects in animal studies, and neither has established human safety. Because the vast majority of human studies have focused on serotonin-specific reuptake inhibitors (SSRIs) and tricyclic antidepressants (TCAs), these drugs are at least well tested. Therefore, SSRIs can be suggested for use during pregnancy, given their better side-effect profile (in pregnant women), if an antidepressant must be given.

Class B antidepressants are bupropion and maprotiline.

Class C antidepressants are SSRIs and monoamino oxidase inhibitors (MAOIs), and other atypical agents (nefazodone, trazodone, mirtazapine, venlafaxine), and all TCAs except those in Class D named below.

Class D: Amitriptyline, imipramine, and nortriptyline.

Which antidepressants have adverse cardiac effects ?

TCAs and trazodone.

Which antidepressants have strong sedative effects?

Amitriptyline, clomipramine, imipramine, mirtazapine, nefazodone, and trazodone.

Which antidepressants have weak or no anticholinergic effects?

SSRIs, bupropion, mirtazapine, nefazodone, trazodone, and venlafaxine. (TCAs and MAOIs have strong anticholinergic effects.)

What is the treatment of choice for atypical depression?

MAOIs (phenelzine, tranylcypromine).

What are the contraindications to bupropion?

Seizure, eating disorders, and use of an MAOI within the previous 14 days.

Facts about MAOIs.

The most common side effect of MAOIs is orthostatic hypotension.

Foods that contain a high level of tyramine (e.g., red wine, aged cheese, nuts, chocolate) are contraindicated during the use of MAOIs.

MAOIs are contraindicated with the use of:

1. All other antidepressants. A 14-day (28-day for fluoxetine) systemic clearance period is necessary.
2. Meperidine.
3. Adrenergic agonists (e.g., phenylephrine, phenylpropanolamine).

Adrenergic antagonists such as phentolamine are not contraindicated with MAOIs.

Lithium is not contraindicated with MAOIs.

What is the clinical presentation of an MAOI-induced hypertensive crisis ?

High blood pressure (BP), headache, stiff neck, and vomiting.

How should an MAOI-induced hypertensive crisis (BP = 240/140 mm Hg with a pounding headache) be treated?

1. The first-choice treatment agent is an α-adrenergic blocking agent given intravenously (IV). Phentolamine (up to 5 mg IV) has been used.
2. Chlorpromazine (25–50 mg intramuscularly [IM] or orally [PO]) can be given as a second-choice agent and is usually available.
3. Oral nifedipine can be given if there is early onset of a severe,

bilateral, pounding occipital headache.

What is the pharmacologic mechanism of action of mirtazapine?

Central α_2-adrenergic receptor antagonism. Since activation of α_2-receptor inhibits the release of serotonin, mirtazapine can increase central serotonergic tone. In addition, mirtazapine blocks 5-hydroxytryptamine types 2 and 3 (5-HT2 and 5-HT3) receptors, and therefore increases the relative activity of 5-HT1A and 5-HT1C receptors.

The sedative effect of mirtazapine is caused by its antagonistic effect at the histamine-1 (H-1) receptor. The sedative effect appears at a low dose, but may <u>weaken at a higher dose.</u>

What are the side effects and drug interactions of nefazodone?

1. <u>Has no anticholinergic effects.</u> (The only antidepressants that have moderate to severe anticholinergic effects are TCAs and MAOIs.)
2. Does not cause sexual dysfunction.
3. Is highly sedative.
4. Is a strong inhibitor of cytochrome P450 <u>3A4.</u> Only triazolam is officially contraindicated for concurrent use with nefazodone.

Benzodiazepines metabolized by P450 3A4 and therefore not recommended for concurrent use with nefazodone are: midazolam, alprazolam, and <u>triazolam</u> (MAT). Diazepam is metabolized by both P450 3A4 and P450 2C19.

What are the characteristics of serotonin syndrome?

It is caused by SSRIs or MAOIs, especially when these are combined with tyramine-containing foods.

The combination of MAOIs with meperidine is contraindicated. A 14-day washout period should be allowed when switching from MAOIs to other antidepressants.

Features of the serotonin syndrome are:

- <u>Jitteriness, myoclonus, tremor at rest, hypertonicity, and rigidity.</u>
- <u>Autonomic instability</u> (diaphoresis, <u>hypo-/hypertension).</u>
- <u>Insomnia,</u> excitement, coma, death.

What are the half-lives of various SSRIs?

Longest: <u>Fluoxetine</u> (7 to 15 days).

Shortest: Fluvoxamine (15 hours).

All other SSRIs: 1 day.

Fluoxetine is the only SSRI with clinically active metabolites (norfluoxetine).

What drug interactions occur with TCAs?

TCAs are metabolized by cytochrome P450 2D6, 1A2, and 3A4.

Cigarette smoking, which induces P450 1A2 , may decrease TCA concentrations.

Some antipsychotic agents (e.g., clozapine, haloperidol, risperidone, thioridazine) are competitors with TCAs for P450 2D6, and therefore increase TCA concentrations.

Methylphenidate decreases the metabolism of TCAs and therefore increases their concentrations.

Drugs that increase TCA levels are antipsychotics and methylphenidate.

Cigarette smoking decreases TCA levels.

What severe reactions have occurred with TCAs?

Cases of sudden death have been reported in children in association with the use of desipramine.

Overdosage with TCAs is associated with arrhythmia, seizure, delirium, and respiratory depression.

What is the best monitoring method to use for a patient who has overdosed on an unknown amount of a TCA?

Electrocardiography.

TCAs can potentially cause cardiac arrhythmia and death.

Which TCA has blood levels that are related to its clinical effect and needs to be monitored?

Nortriptyline.

The clinical therapeutic blood level for nortriptyline is 50–150 ng/mL.

What are the major effects and properties of venlafaxine?

Venlafaxine blocks reuptake of three neurotransmitters: serotonin, norepinephrine, and dopamine.

It may cause increased diastolic BP.

Its half-life is very short among antidepressants (5 hours, and the half-life of its metabolite, desmethylvenlafaxine, 12 hours).

Venlafaxine does not inhibit cytochrome P450.

What are the half-lives of various benzodiazepines?

Short (hours): Triazolam (Halcion), oxazepam (Serax). Benzodiazepines with short half-lives are associated with rebound insomnia when their use is discontinued.

Intermediate (< 1 day): Alprazolam (Xanax), lorazepam (Ativan).

Long (> 1 day): Clonazepam (Klonopin)

Very long (days): <u>Diazepam</u> (Valium), chlordiazepoxide (Librium).

What benzodiazepines are safe to use in patients with compromised hepatic function?

<u>Temazepam,</u> oxazepam, and lorazepam. These drugs do not need oxidation, and have no active metabolites.

TOL (temazepam, oxazepam, and lorazepam).

What is the mechanism of action of benzodiazepines?

Benzodiazepines bind to binding sites (also known as <u>benzodiazepine receptors</u>) on receptors for γ-aminobutyric acid (GABA) and <u>enhance the effects of GABA.</u>

Benzodiazepine receptors are not independent receptors. They are specific binding sites located on GABA receptors.

Which benzodiazepines are available in parenteral form?

Four benzodiazepines have parenteral forms:

1. Chlordiazepoxide: Has multiple active metabolites (including diazepam), a medium rate of absorption, and a long duration of action.
2. Diazepam: Has multiple active metabolites, a rapid rate of

absorption, and a long duration of action.

3. Lorazepam: Has no active metabolites, <u>a reliably rapid-to-medium rate of absorption,</u> and a short duration of action.

4. Midazolam: This drug is available for IV injection, has active metabolites, and has a short duration of action.

What is the drug of first choice in the treatment of catatonia?

A benzodiazepine. The most commonly used agent is lorazepam (Ativan) given IM.

What are the major differences in side-effect profiles of typical low-potency and typical high-potency antipsychotic agents?

Low-potency agents are more likely to cause hypotension, anticholinergic effects, and sedation, and less likely to cause extrapyramidal side effects (EPS).

High-potency agents are more likely to cause EPS and less likely to cause hypotension, anticholinergic effects, and sedation.

Commonly used typical antipsychotic agents:

High potency: <u>Haloperidol (Haldol),</u> fluphenazine (Prolixin).

Medium potency: Molindone (Moban), loxapine (Loxitane).

Low potency: <u>Chlorpromazine</u> (Thorazine), thiothixene (Navane).

Elderly persons are more sensitive to <u>anticholinergic effects,</u> and may become confused when given an antipsychotic agent.

What are the treatment modalities for neuroleptic malignant syndrome (NMS)?

Discontinue antipsychotics, <u>hydration</u> (IV fluids), <u>cooling,</u> dantrolene, and <u>bromocriptine</u> (Parlodel).

What are anticholinergic effects?

Symptoms: <u>Dryness of the mouth, urinary retention, decreased bronchial secretion, tachycardia, and constipation. Memory impairment</u> may occur at toxic doses.

Treatment: <u>Bethanechol</u> (Urecholine), or reduce anticholinergic drug dosage.

Psychiatric medicines with anticholinergic effects are:

1. Among antipsychotic agents: <u>clozapine</u> (Clozaril), <u>thioridazine</u> (Navane), and mesoridazine (Serentil) have strong anticholinergic effects. All other antipsychotic agents have weak cholinergic effects.
2. Among antidepressants, <u>TCAs</u> and MAOIs have strong anticholinergic effects. All other

antidepressants have weak anticholinergic effects.

Other drugs that have anticholinergic effects include antiparkinsonian agents such as benztropine (Cogentin).

What is the side-effect profile of clozapine?

The most common side effect is sedation.

Important severe reactions are seizures, agranulocytosis, and NMS.

Other common side effects are hypotension, headache, hyperglycemia, and weight gain.

Clozapine has a minimum effect on prolactin level.

What are the clinical features of NMS?

General: Altered consciousness, fever, and mutism.

Autonomic: Labile blood pressure, tachycardia, diaphoresis, incontinence, dysphasia.

Muscular: Rigidity, tremor.

Hematologic: Leukocytosis, elevated creatine kinase.

What is the mechanism by which NMS occurs?

Blockade of dopamine receptors in the basal ganglia, hypothalamus, postganglionic sympathetic neurons, and smooth muscle. NMS may also involve blockade of non-dopamine monoamines.

Besides being caused by typical antipsychotic agents, NMS may also be caused by TCA, SSRI, and atypical antipsychotic agents.

The risk of NMS is increased with use of lithium and sudden discontinuation of levodopa.

What are the important drug interactions of carbamazepine?

Carbamazepine induces liver enzymes that increases its own metabolism and may also reduce the effectiveness of other medicines such as oral contraceptives. As a result of this effect, the serum level of carbamazepine may drop over a period of months. Periodic reassessment of the carbamazepine serum level is therefore necessary, and its dosage should be adjusted accordingly.

The concentration of carbamazepine is increased with concurrent use of cimetidine.

Liver-enzyme-induction: Carbamazepine.

Liver-enzyme-inhibition: Cimetidine.

What are the important drug interactions of lithium?

Drugs that increase lithium levels are angiotensin converting enzyme inhibitors, fluoxetine, ibuprofen (Motrin), indomethacin (Indocin), and diuretics (spironolactone, thiazide).

Drugs that decrease lithium levels are theophylline, caffeine, and laxatives.

What are the effects of lithium intoxication?

Cardiac: ST-segment depression and QT-interval prolongation on the electrocardiogram.

Neuromuscular: Ataxia, coarse tremor, dysarthria, and epilepsy.

Kidney: Nephrotoxicity (interstitial fibrosis).

Thyroid: None. Lithium may cause hypothyroidism. This is a side effect that remits when lithium is discontinued. Lithium is not thyrotoxic.

Treatment: Supportive; hemodialysis if the serum lithium level is above 4.0 mmol/L.

What are the mechanisms of action of lithium?

1. Lithium does not work at the synapse through effects of neurotransmitters.

2. Lithium works at the level of G-proteins and other second messengers, such as phosphatidylinositol phosphate (PIP).

Current hypotheses: Lithium blocks the G-protein-mediated transmission of messages through:

1. Inhibition of inositol monophosphate phosphatase (IMPase).
2. Inhibition of the alpha unit of G-proteins.
3. Inhibition of glycogen synthase kinase-3β (GSK-3β).
4. Inhibition of adenylyl cyclase.

How is lithium metabolized?

Lithium is not metabolized, and its half-life does not change with impaired hepatic function. Lithium is excreted via the kidney.

What are the side effects of lithium?

1. Tremor: This may occur at therapeutic levels of lithium. Treatment involves dividing the dose, reducing coffee intake, or uses of a β-blocker (propranolol).
2. Polyuria/polydipsia (nephrogenic diabetes insipidus): Is treated with amiloride, a potassium-sparing diuretic that inhibits sodium

resorption at the distal convoluted tubule.

3. Weight gain: Caused by increased caloric intake.

4. Hypothyroidism: Lithium inhibits iodine uptake, iodination of tyrosine, and the release of triiodothyronine (T3) and thyroxine (T4).

5. Rash.

Lithium has no adverse effects on the respiratory system.

What factors are important in maintenance treatment with lithium?

A dramatic change in the sodium serum concentration may change the serum lithium concentration. It is important to maintain usual sodium and fluid intake during lithium treatment.

Massive fluid shifts (pregnancy/labor) may change lithium concentrations.

Close monitoring of lithium levels is required in patients with unstable renal function or congestive heart disease.

Which psychiatric medicine may cause nephrogenic diabetes insipidus (DI)?

Lithium. DI is not associated with other psychiatric medicines.

Please note that the syndrome of inappropriate secretion of antidiuretic hormone (SIADH) is associated with many psychiatric medicines.

DI: Lack of antidiuretic hormone (ADH), also known as vasopressin, or a poor renal response to ADH. SIADH is marked by an abnormally high level of ADH.

ADH acts at the renal collecting tubules to enhance free-water resorption.

Which thyroid function test should be repeated at 6 months for patients taking lithium?

Thyroid-stimulating hormone (TSH).

What is the treatment of choice for rapidly cycling mood disorder?

Anticonvulsant agents, such as valproic acid.

What are the side effects of valproic acid?

Common: Weight gain, <u>hair loss.</u>

Less common: <u>Thrombocytopenia,</u> bone-marrow suppression.

Congenital defects: <u>Neural tube,</u> cardiac, limb, and facial, and hypospadias.

Hirsutism: Phenytoin.

Hair loss: Valproic acid.

What laboratory test is needed in carbamazepine-treated patients at 2-week intervals during the first 2 months of treatment?

A <u>complete blood count (CBC)</u> for the early detection of blood dyscrasias, such as aplastic anemia, agranulocytosis, leukopenia, and thrombocytopenia.

Also, liver function tests to detect drug-induced hepatitis.

What medicines have inhibitory effects on cytochrome P450 enzymes?

<u>Nefazodone,</u> fluvoxamine and TCAs: High inhibition of P450 3A4.

Sertraline, fluoxetine: Low inhibition of P450 3A4.

<u>Paroxetine,</u> fluoxetine: High inhibition of P450 2D6

TCAs, sertraline: Low inhibition of P450 2D6.

Benzodiazepines metabolized by P450 3A4 are midazolam, alprazolam, and triazolam.

Diazepam is metabolized by both P450 3A4 and P450 2C19.

Triazolam (Halcion) is contraindicated for concurrent use with nefazodone.

Which drugs cause drug-induced delayed ejaculation and retrograde ejaculation?

Drugs with α-adrenergic antagonistic effects. Most typical antipsychotics have significant antagonistic effects on α-adrenergic receptors. Drugs known to have such side effects include <u>thioridazine</u> and chlorpromazine.

What are the causes of extrapyramidal symptoms (EPS), and how are they treated?

Mechanisms: EPS are theoretically attributed to <u>blockage of dopamine-2 (D2) receptors in the nigrostriatal pathway,</u> and to these receptors' subsequent supersensitivity.

Treatment:

Akathisia: <u>Propranolol.</u>

Acute dystonia: Benztropine (Cogentin) or diphenhydramine (Benadryl).

What are the core features of neuroleptic-induced dystonia?

Abnormal positioning or spasm of the muscles of the head, neck, limbs, or trunk, developing within a few days of starting a neuroleptic medication or raising its dose.

Neuroleptic-induced parkinsonism is marked by a parkinsonian tremor, muscular rigidity, or akinesia developing within a few <u>weeks</u> of starting a neuroleptic medication or raising its dose.

Neuroleptic-induced akathisia is marked by subjective complaints of restlessness accompanied by observed movements (e.g., fidgety movements of the legs, rocking from foot to foot, pacing, or inability to sit or stand still) developing within a few <u>weeks</u> of starting a *neuroleptic medication or raising its dose.*

Neuroleptic-induced tardive dyskinesia is marked by involuntary choreiform, athetoid, or rhythmic movements (lasting at least a few weeks) of the tongue, jaw, or extremities and developing in association with the use of neuroleptic medication for at least a few <u>months.</u>

What is meperidine?

An analgesic agent.

Meperidine may cause seizure, contraindicated with use of MAOIs.

COGENTIN

What are the symptoms of benztropine intoxication?

Crazy: <u>Agitation,</u> hallucinations.

Dry: Dry skin, <u>dry mouth.</u>

Red: Flushing, hyperthermia.

Hypotension, tachycardia, mydriasis (<u>dilated pupils</u>), decreased bowel sounds, seizure, delirium, and coma.

Which typical antipsychotic agent is least likely to cause weight gain?

Molindone (Moban).

What is the mechanism of orthostatic hypotension?

Blockade of α_1-adrenergic receptors.

What psychiatric medications cause priapism?

Priapism is a rare but important side effect of <u>trazodone.</u>

Other medicines that may cause priapism include venlafaxine, levodopa, and sildenafil.

Retinal pigmentation is an adverse effect of which antipsychotic agent?

Retinal pigmentation may be associated with the use of <u>thioridazine</u> (Mellaril) at high doses (above 800 mg/day).

What are some risk factors for tardive dyskinesia?

Old age, mood disorder, <u>female gender,</u> childhood, <u>African-American heritage</u>, and diabetes.

What are some indications for psychostimulants?

AD/HD.

Narcolepsy.

Exogenous obesity.

Depression in elderly and medically ill persons.

Psychostimulants should <u>not</u> be used in <u>personality disorders</u> or for patients with a history of substance abuse.

What are the choices of pharmacologic treatment for attention-deficit/hyperactivity disorder (AD/HD)?

<u>Stimulants:</u> Methylphenidate (Ritalin) is usually the drug of first choice. Dextroamphetamine (Dexedrine) and amphetamine (Adderall) may be used as drugs of first choice or alternatives. Pemoline (Cylert) may cause liver failure.

Antidepressants: <u>Bupropion</u> (Wellbutrin) and other antidepressants.

Clonidine.

How are beta-blockers used in psychiatry?

Beta-blockers have been less frequently used in psychiatric treatment in recent years than formerly. They are still useful in the treatment of social phobia. They are also used to reduce or reverse side effects caused by other psychopharmacologic treatment, such as <u>lithium-induced postural tremor</u> and neuroleptic-induced acute akathisia.

Tagamet

What drug interactions occur with cimetidine?

Cimetidine inhibits liver enzymes, and increases the serum concentration of many drugs, including:

<u>SSRIs.</u>

Benzodiazepines.

Anticonvulsants (<u>carbamazepine,</u> phenytoin, valproic acid derivatives).

Beta-blockers.

TCAs.

Sildenafil (Viagra).

What is the first-pass effect?	Initial metabolism of a drug within the <u>portal circulation</u> of the liver before the drugs reach the systemic circulation.
What are some metabolic characteristics of geriatric patients?	Increased <u>fat.</u> Decreased <u>hepatic metabolism,</u> intestinal motility, <u>plasma-binding proteins (albumin), glomerular filtration rate,</u> and renal clearance.
What pharmacologic treatment is available for obsessive, compulsive disorder (OCD)?	Antidepressants with serotonergic effects, such as <u>SSRIs, clomipramine, and MAOIs.</u> High doses are needed. Antidepressants without serotonergic effects, such as <u>bupropion,</u> are not effective.
How is seasonal depression diagnosed and treated?	Seasonal depression in diagnosed with the *Diagnostic and Statistical Manual of the American Psychiatric Association, Fourth Revision,* by applying a seasonal pattern specifier to major depressive disorder or bipolar disorders. The treatment for seasonal depression is <u>phototherapy.</u>
What are the indications for electroconvulsive therapy (ECT)?	Well-established indications for ECT are: <u>Catatonia,</u> MDD, mania, and schizophrenia (acute psychosis). Other indications: Delirium, OCD, seizure, and Parkinson's disease.

ECT is not effective in: <u>somatization disorder,</u> personality disorders, anxiety disorders.

ECT is usually not effective in: <u>chronic schizophrenia.</u>

Absolute contraindications: None.

Relative contraindications: Cardiovascular conditions, space-occupying intracerebral lesions, cerebral aneurysms, recent strokes.

What are the mechanisms of action of ECT?

They are unknown. The assumed primary therapeutic component is the <u>bilateral spread of convulsion.</u>

What medicines should be discontinued before ECT is given?

Lithium and benzodiazepines.

What are the side effects of ECT?

1. Headache.
2. Confusion: Up to 10% of patients experience confusion within 30 minutes after treatment; this usually resolves spontaneously.
3. Delirium: This typically clears within days.
4. Memory impairment: <u>No permanent brain damage.</u> Almost <u>all patients recover</u> to baseline memory status after 6 months.

5. Cardiac arrhythmias: Mild and transient, occurring more commonly in patients with cardiac disease. Usually induced by postictal <u>vagal hyperactivity</u> that causes bradycardia.

6. <u>High blood pressure:</u> Blood pressure increases transiently during seizures. *Noempanil Panada*

Which psychiatric drugs require routine monitoring of their serum levels?

Lithium, desipramine, nortriptyline, valproic acid, and carbamazepine.

What medications are effective for the treatment of panic disorder?

1 Benzodiazepines.

2 TCAs.

3 MAOIs.

4 SSRIs.

What was the first psychiatric medicine to be introduced into clinical use?

<u>Chlorpromazine</u> (Thorazine), introduced in 1953.

Other landmark agents in psychopharmacology:

First mood stabilizer: Lithium, introduced in 1949.

First antidepressant: TCAs, particularly Tofranil, introduced in 1957.

First SSRI: Fluoxetine (Prozac), introduced in 1985.

Withdrawal from what substance may cause grand mal seizure as well as severe anxiety and insomnia?

Alcohol.

Benzodiazepines.

Barbiturates.

Meprobamate.

Eq values *Meprobamate is a nonbenzodiazepine anxiolytic agent with muscle-relaxant properties.*

What pharmacologic agents are usually used to manage acute violent episodes in the emergency department setting?

Haloperidol and benzodiazepine.

Chapter 15 Neurology

A 5-year-old child was observed to suddenly stop all activities for several seconds, and to blink his eyes. No confusion was found. What is the probable diagnosis?

Absence seizures, also known as "petit mal seizure."

Summary of absence seizures:

1. Age: Begin in <u>childhood.</u> Usually do not persist after age 20 years.
2. Induction: Hyperventilation.
3. Presentations: <u>Brief loss of consciousness, no loss of postural tone,</u> subtle motor manifestations (<u>eye blinking,</u> head turning), and rare automatisms.
4. Recovery: <u>Immediate recovery</u> with full orientation.
5. Treatment: Ethosuximide (Zarontin) and valproic acid. LMT6

Valproic acid is also indicated for treating generalized tonic–clonic, myoclonic, and partial seizures.

When should anticoagulants be used in cerebral vascular diseases?

Indicated in cases of transient ischemic attack (TIA) and completed stroke with a cardiac source.

Consider in: Stroke in evolution, TIA, or completed stroke with a carotid or vertebrobasilar artery source.

What is the cause of benign intracranial hypertension?

The cause is unknown, but this condition may be associated with <u>vitamin A intoxication.</u>

What are the characteristic features of narcolepsy?

Sudden onset of sleep with loss of muscle tone, in association with emotional stress or physical exertion.

What is the treatment of choice for nocturnal myoclonic sleep disorder?

Benzodiazepines.

What are the pathologic characteristics of Pick's disease?

1. Prominent frontotemporal atrophy.
2. Neuron cell inclusions: Clustered cytoskeletal elements.
3. Early personality and behavioral changes.
4. Other cognitive functions are relatively preserved.

What are the pathologic characteristics of Wilson's disease?

<u>Psychosis and liver dysfunction.</u> Other symptoms include a Kayer-Fleischer (K-F) ring on the cornea, dysarthria, tremor, poor coordination, dystonia, and hypersexuality.

Treatment: Avoidance of copper-rich foods; use of <u>penicillamine,</u> potassium sulfide, pyridoxine, and zinc acetate.

What are the clinical findings in chronic subdural hematoma?

Initial symptom: Headache.

Common symptoms: Altered mental status, confusion, <u>cognitive dysfunction,</u> hemiparesis, papilledema, and extensor plantar responses.

<u>Focal symptoms often appear later</u> than global symptoms.

What is "locked-in syndrome?"

A result of functional transection of the brain stem below the mid-pons. Such patients are <u>mute and quadriplegic, but do not lose consciousness,</u> because the reticular formation lies above the level of the mid-pons. <u>Eye movement is intact.</u>

Causes include infarct, hemorrhage, myelinolysis, tumor, and encephalitis.

What is Wallenberg's syndrome?

Lateral medullary infarction. The clinical features vary, depending on the extent of infarction.

Structures affected and the corresponding clinical features are:

1. <u>Vestibular nuclei: Vertigo, nystagmus.</u>
2. <u>Inferior cerebellar peduncle: Hemiataxia.</u>
3. Spinal tract and nucleus of trigeminal nerve: Impairment of

sensory modalities over the face.

4. Descending sympathetic tract: Ipsilateral Horner's syndrome.

5. Spinothalamic tract: Loss of light and position sense in the ipsilateral limbs, impairment of pinprick and temperature sensation in the contralateral limbs.

6. Dorsal motor nucleus of the vagus nerve: Nausea, vomiting, dysphagia, and hoarseness.

What is temporary hemianopsia and what is its most common cause?

Temporary loss of vision in one half of the visual field of one or both eyes. Commonly caused by migraine.

What are the characteristics of ulnar nerve dysfunction?

The ulnar nerve is particularly susceptible to mechanical injury at the elbow by adjacent anatomic structures. This is also known as "ulnar nerve entrapment."

Clinical presentations include: Pain, <u>sensory loss, and weakness in the fourth and fifth fingers and the ulnar border of the hand.</u>

After a motor-vehicle accident, the victim had no obvious open trauma and no loss of consciousness, and behaved normally. However, 30 minutes after the accident, he turned pale, and lost consciousness, and collapsed. <u>He recovered completely within minutes.</u> What is the most likely diagnosis?

Vasovagal syncope. The key to this diagnosis is rapid recovery after assumption of the horizontal position.

If the patient had not recovered within a few minutes, a subdural hematoma should have been considered.

What are the signs of a poor prognosis in Bell's palsy?

Severe pain and <u>complete palsy.</u>

What is the mechanism of action of carbidopa in the treatment of Parkinson's disease?

<u>Blockade of peripheral dopa decarboxylase,</u> augmenting the action of levodopa.

What brain tumors are common in children but rare in adults?

Medulloblastoma.

What brain tumors are common in adults but rare in children?

Glioblastoma multiforme, metastatic tumors.

What brain tumors are common in both children and adults?

Astrocytoma (more common in children).

What are the electrophysiologic signs of muscle denervation?

Fibrillations, positive sharp waves.

What are the side effects of phenytoin (Dilantin)?

Dose-related side effects are: Diplopia, ataxia, gingival hyperplasia, hirsutism, coarse facial features, polyneuropathy, osteomalacia, and megaloblastic anemia.

Idiosyncratic side effects are: Skin rash, fever, lymphoid hyperplasia, hepatic dysfunction, blood dyscrasia, and Stevens–Johnson syndrome.

Hirsutism: Phenytoin
Hair loss: Valproic acid

What is the drug of choice for the treatment of psychotic symptoms in Parkinson's disease?

Clozapine was once the only choice. Recent reports support olanzapine and quetiapine. The choice among these three agents should be based on clinical judgment.

What pharmacological treatments are used for migraine?

Acute treatment: Non-narcotic analgesics, prochlorperazine, ergotamine, dihydroergotamine, and sumatriptan (Imitrex).

Prophylaxis: Tricyclic antidepressants (amitriptyline, nortriptyline), low-dose ergot preparations, methysergide, valproate, calcium–channel antagonists (verapamil, nifedipine).

What are the pathognomonic features of subarachnoid hemorrhage?

Sudden <u>severe headache, relative preservation of consciousness,</u> lack of focal signs, <u>neck stiffness.</u> Possible collapse.

A statement of "the worst headache in my life" is not necessary.

What is internuclear ophthalmoplegia?

Internuclear ophthalmoplegia presents as disconjugate gaze with impaired adduction and nystagmus of the abducted eye.

When the patient attempts to look to the left, the left eye turns to the left with nystagmus, and the right eye cannot turn to the left, and vice versa when the patient attempts to look to the right.

The location of the lesion in internuclear ophthalmoplegia is the medial longitudinal fasciculus.

Most common causes: In young adults, multiple sclerosis; in older patients, vascular diseases.

Gaze right (Fig. 1).

Gaze left (Fig. 2)

What are the clinical features of diabetic ophthalmoplegia?

Isolated impairments from an isolated lesion of the oculomotor, trochlear, or abducens nerve, not seen in a computed tomography (CT) or magnetic resonance imaging (MRI) scan.

Pupillary sparing: Infarction of the central portion of the oculomotor nerve with sparing of the peripheral fibers that mediate pupillary regulation.

Vision is impaired in one eye. When light is shone in the healthy eye, both pupils react.

In optic neuritis, the affected eye shows a diminished pupillary reaction to light.

What are the characteristics of carpal tunnel syndrome?

Compression of the median nerve caused by:

Myxedema (from hypothyroidism).
Pregnancy.
Trauma or other sources.

Pain and sensory deficits (paresthesias) of the palmar surface are confined to a median nerve distribution (i.e., involving primarily the thumb, index, and middle fingers and the lateral half of the ring finger).

Weakness in abduction of the thumb.

Possible pain in the arm.

What is benign positional vertigo?

Etiology:

Peripheral: Canalolithiasis.

Central: Unknown.

Symptoms:

- <u>Brief, severe vertigo with nausea and vomiting upon changes in head position,</u> most severe in the lateral decubitus position with the affected ear facing down.
- Persistence of vertigo for several weeks followed by its spontaneous resolution.
- No hearing loss.
- Positional nystagmus always accompanying vertigo and typically unidirectional, rotatory, and delayed in onset by several seconds after assumption of the precipitating head position.
- Nystagmus and vertigo inducible by rapid movement from a sitting to a recumbent position with the head 45 degrees below the horizontal plane. This is called the Dix–Hallpike maneuver. <u>Repetition of this maneuver can attenuate the response.</u>

Treatment: Repositioning maneuvers.

Of what disease is involuntary gait acceleration a characteristic feature?

Parkinson's disease.

What are the features of gait in Parkinson's disease?

Postural instability and a tendency to accelerate involuntarily with small steps. The patient walks with rigid, shuffling steps and a narrow base. There is a tendency to lean forward to accelerate the speed of walking.

What visual impairment may present in the case of a lesion in the optic tract?

Contralateral homonymous hemianopsia. The optic tract is connected to the ipsilateral retina, which reflects the contralateral visual field (Fig. 3).

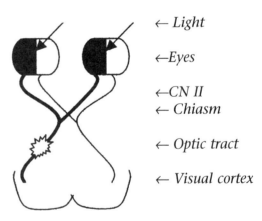

← Light

←Eyes

←CN II
← Chiasm

← Optic tract

← Visual cortex

What is the type of tremor characteristic of Parkinson's disease?

Rest tremor, or tremor is prominent in the resting state, and attenuated during voluntary movement (e.g., when the patient attempts to do the finger–nose–finger test).

How is pseudoseizure distinguished from genuine seizure?

In pseudoseizure there is:

1. No tonic phase (e.g., <u>no synchronous limb thrashing</u>).
2. No real loss of consciousness or <u>behavioral automatism,</u> although there may be apparent "loss of consciousness."
3. <u>No postictal confusion.</u>
4. <u>No urinary incontinence.</u>
5. No seizure activity in the electroencephalogram (EEG).

Which comorbid diseases of acquired immunodeficiency syndrome (AIDS) produce cerebral focal lesions?

Toxoplasmosis and lymphoma.

What cerebral areas are often involved in closed-head contusions with loss of consciousness?

The bases of the frontal lobes and the tips of the temporal lobes.

Classification of seizures:

1. Generalized seizures:
   A. <u>Tonic–clonic</u> (grand mal).
   B. <u>Absence</u> (petit mal).
   C. Other (tonic, clonic, <u>myoclonic</u>).
2. Partial seizures:
   A. Simple partial.
   B. Complex partial (temporal lobe, psychomotor).

Jacksonian seizure:

Also called "Jacksonian march." A simple partial seizure that may spread (march) to contiguous regions of the motor cortex.

What visual lesion is likely to be caused by a pituitary tumor?

Bitemporal hemianopia (Fig. 4).

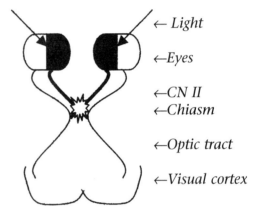

← *Light*

←*Eyes*

←*CN II*
←*Chiasm*

←*Optic tract*

←*Visual cortex*

What are the clinical features of myasthenia gravis?

1. Insidious onset. Slowly progressive course.
2. Diplopia, ptosis, dysarthria, extremity weakness, generalized weakness, dysphagia.
3. Weakness does not conform to the distribution of any single nerve.
4. Pupillary responses are not affected.
5. Persistent activity of a muscle group leads to temporarily increased weakness, <u>with restoration of strength after a brief rest.</u>

What are the clinical findings in cases of upper-motor-neuron lesions?

1. Weakness/paralysis, spasticity.
2. Increased tendon reflexes, positive (pathologic) Babinski's reflex.
3. No significant muscle atrophy.

What is subacute combined degeneration and how is it treated?

1. Symptoms: Distal paresthesias, absent reflexes, weakness, loss of proprioception, spastic paraparesis, positive Babinski's sign, ataxia, and dementia.
2. Cause: Vitamin B_{12} deficiency (pernicious anemia, gastrointestinal surgery, sprue, fish tapeworm, and strict vegetarian diet).
3. Diagnostic tests: Serum vitamin B_{12} assay, Schilling test.
4. Treatment: Intramuscular administration of vitamin B_{12}.

A patient develops progressive weakness 2 weeks after a viral infection. What is the possible diagnosis and what laboratory test can be used to prove it?

Guillain–Barré syndrome (acute idiopathic inflammatory polyneuropathy).

Clinical presentation:

1. Symmetric weakness, usually beginning in the legs, and more marked proximally than distally.
2. Some sensory complaints.
3. Typical absence of deep tendon reflexes. There may be marked autonomic dysfunction.

4. Slow conduction velocity and prolonged distal motor latency in and conduction block in nerve conduction studies.
5. Cerebrospinal fluid (CSF) shows an increased protein concentration but a normal cell count. Electrophysiologic study shows marked slowing of motor- and sensory-nerve conduction velocity, indicating denervation and axonal loss.

Treatment: plasmapheresis, intravenous immunoglobulin.

What are the critical diagnostic features of Guillain–Barré syndrome (acute idiopathic inflammatory polyneuropathy)?

1. Acute onset (days).
2. Progressive and relatively symmetric weakness.
3. Absent tendon reflexes.
4. CSF shows an elevated protein concentration and white cell count ≤ 10/μL.
5. Nerve conduction study shows conduction block.

What is Brown–Séquard syndrome?

A syndrome that results from hemisection of the spinal cord. Below the level of the lesion, the patient has an ipsilateral deficit in motor, vibration, and joint-position sense, and a contralateral loss of pain and temperature sense.

Is the direction of eye deviation during a seizure related to the location of the seizure focus?

EEG studies have shown that the location of a seizure focus is related to the direction of eye deviation. During a seizure, the eyes deviate in the direction of the seizure focus. Postictally, the eyes deviate away from the seizure focus.

The patient looks in the direction of the excited neuron.

What is the most effective treatment for focal dystonia?

Botulinum toxin.

Examples of focal dystonia are blepharospasm, oromandibular dystonia, spasmodic torticollis, and writer's cramp.

How does botulinum toxin work in the treatment of blepharospasm, dystonic dysphonia, and torticollis?

It prevents the release of acetylcholine vesicles from presynaptic nerve terminals. In this way it reduces muscle spasm.

How does vertigo differ from syncope?

Vertigo is the illusion of movement of the body or the environment. It is caused by lesions affecting the labyrinth of the inner ear, the vestibular division of the auditory nerve, or brain-stem vestibular nuclei.

Syncope results from the impaired brain supply of blood, oxygen, or glucose.

A 29-year-old woman complains of vertigo and diplopia. Physical examination finds that when she looks to the left, she has nystagmus of the left eye only, with failure of adduction of the right eye. The manifestation pattern of ocular motility in this case suggests the diagnosis of what disease?

Multiple sclerosis.

This is a typical presentation of internuclear ophthalmoplegia. If the patient were elderly, with symptoms of new onset, the differential diagnosis would include vascular diseases.

What are characteristic CSF findings in multiple sclerosis?

Oligoclonal bands of immunoglobulin G and myelin basic protein on protein electrophoresis.

What is amyotrophic lateral sclerosis?

It is a mixed upper- and lower-motor-neuron deficit found in the limbs, although there may also be bulbar involvement of the upper- or lower-motor-neuron type.

The limb involvement in ALS is characterized by easy fatigability, weakness, stiffness, twitching, wasting, and muscle cramping.

There may be vague sensory complaints and weight loss, but examination shows no sensory deficit.

Physical examination shows <u>atrophy of the intrinsic muscles</u> and <u>brisk reflexes</u>. Electrophysiologic study shows <u>widespread fasciculations</u> and fibrillations, and positive sharp waves.

What is the cerebral location for olfactory hallucinations followed by altered consciousness and orofacial automatisms?

Anterior medial temporal lobe.

What is the treatment of choice for the abnormal involuntary movement associated with Huntington's chorea?

<u>Haloperidol,</u> chlorpromazine, or reserpine (a dopamine-depleting agent).

Huntington's chorea:

Typical features: Dementia and chorea, with a positive family history.

Molecular mechanism: Expansion of CAG trinucleotide repeat sequences at chromosome 4p16.3.

What is the major ocular symptom of carotid insufficiency?

Transient monocular blindness.

What is typical gait in alcoholic cerebellar degeneration?

The patient walks with poor balance, reeling, and on a broad base. Steps are variable in length and poorly coordinated. Balance is poor with the eyes open or closed.

What language deficiency is typical in a stroke in the inferior frontal convolution, caused by occlusion of the anterior branches of the left middle cerebral artery?

Impaired fluency of spontaneous speech (Broca's aphasia)

What are the characteristics and treatment of pseudotumor cerebri (benign intracranial hypertension)?

Symptoms: <u>Headache, papilledema, and diminished visual acuity.</u>

Evaluation: MRI or CT shows either normal or typical small (slitlike) ventricles and <u>increased intracranial pressure.</u>

Pseudotumor cerebri is more common in <u>women</u> than in men, and reaches a peak frequency in the <u>third decade.</u>

Treatment: Acetazolamide (a carbonic anhydrase inhibitor).

What are the contraindications to the use of tissue plasminogen activator (TPA) for thrombolysis in acute stroke?

Risk of hemorrhage including:

- Prior intracranial hemorrhage.
- Seizure at the onset of stroke symptoms.
- Stroke or trauma occurring less than 3 months before the presenting stroke.
- A major surgical procedure within 14 days.

- Gastrointestinal or urinary tract bleeding within 21 days.
- Systolic blood pressure (BP) over 185 mmHg or diastolic BP over 110 mmHg.
- Current treatment with coumadin for atrial fibrillation.

To avoid unnecessary treatment:

- When neurologic deficits are improving rapidly and spontaneously.
- When deficits are mild and isolated.
- In the presence of hypo- or hyperglycemia (which can cause symptoms mimicking a stroke).
- When symptoms have begun more than 3 hours before the proposed TPA therapy.

The patient's clinical symptoms (change in consciousness, headache, agitation, etc.) are usually not influential factors in the decision to undertake TPA treatment.

What MRI finding is characteristic of multi-infarct dementia?

Multiple areas of increased T2-weighted density in the periventricular area.

What measures should be taken to assess hearing loss?

Normal:

Weber's test: Sound perceived as coming from the midline.

Rinne's test: Air conduction more rapid than bone conduction.

Sensorineural hearing loss:

Weber's test: Sound perceived as coming from the normal ear.

Rinne's test: Air conduction more rapid than bone conduction.

Conduction hearing loss:

Weber's test: Sound perceived as coming from the affected ear.

Rinne's test: Bone conduction more rapid than air conduction on the affected side.

Weber's test: A high-pitched (512 Hz) tuning fork is struck and the handle placed on the midline of the patient's forehead. If there is conductive loss, the tone will sound louder in the affected ear; if the loss is sensorineural, the tone will be louder in the unaffected ear.

Rinne's test: The base of a lightly vibrating high-pitched (512 Hz) tuning fork is placed on the mastoid process until the patient no longer perceives the sound, and the still-vibrating fork is then brought up close to (not touching) the ear. Normally—or if the hearing loss is sensorineural—air conduction is greater than bone conduction and the patient will again hear the tone. If there is significant conductive loss, the patient will not be able to hear the air-conducted tone longer than the bone-conducted tone.

What procedure should be chosen to diagnose spinal-cord compression?

MRI.

What is the treatment for trigeminal neuralgia (tic douloureux)?

Carbamazepine can induce remission of symptoms in 24 hours. Phenytoin will abort an acute attack.

What is the most significant risk factor for primary intracerebral hemorrhage?

Hypertension.

Involuntary jerking of the legs while falling asleep that is not associated with discomfort and ceases during sleep is most likely to be what?

A normal phenomenon without pathologic significance.

What vitamin, taken before conception, can reduce the incidence of neural tube defects, such as myelomeningocele?

Folic acid.

It is recommended that pregnant female patients who take valproic acid take folic acid.

What is transient global amnesia?

It is a syndrome of <u>acute memory loss</u> that tends to occur in <u>middle-aged or elderly patients.</u> It is primarily a disorder of short-term memory, and typically lasts for hours.

Patients with transient global amnesia appear agitated and perplexed, and <u>repeatedly inquire about their whereabouts,</u> the time, and the nature of what they are experiencing.

Knowledge of personal identity is preserved, as are remote memories and registration.

The patient's obvious concern about the condition distinguishes transient global amnesia from other organically based amnestic syndromes and psychogenic amnesia.

What are the causes, effects, and diagnostic findings in hypertensive encephalopathy?

A sudden increase in blood pressure may result in encephalopathy and <u>headache</u> in hours to days.

<u>Vomiting,</u> visual disturbances, focal neurologic deficits, and focal or <u>generalized seizures</u> can occur.

<u>Coexisting renal failure</u> increases the risk of this disorder.

Retinal arteriolar spasm is almost invariably present. <u>Papilledema, retinal hemorrhages,</u> and exudates are usually present.

<u>A CT scan</u> or MRI T2-weighted study shows <u>low-density areas</u> suggestive of <u>edema</u> in the <u>posterior regions of the hemispheric white matter.</u>

T1-weighted images are used for optimal visualization of normal anatomy.

T2-weighted images are used to detect areas of pathology.

What are the clinical features of complex partial epilepsy of temporal lobe origin?

Consciousness is <u>impaired but not lost.</u>

Epigastric sensations are most common, but affective (fear), cognitive (déjà vu), and sensory (olfactory hallucinations) may occur.

Seizures generally last for less than 30 minutes (average: 1 to 3 minutes).

The motor manifestation of complex partial epilepsy is termed "automatism," which takes the form of orobuccolingual movements in about 75% of patients and other facial or neck movements in about 50%.

What is the most frequent cause of dementia in the United States?

Alzheimer's disease.

What is the characteristic EEG pattern of hepatic encephalopathy?

Large, bilaterally synchronous triphasic slow waves.

Some other EEG patterns:

Absence seizure: A spike-and-wave pattern that occurs at a frequency of 3 cycles/sec.

Normal adult drowsiness: Frontocentral beta activity may become more prominent.

Stage I sleep: High-voltage single or complex theta or delta waves appearing centrally.

What does a positive Romberg's test indicate?

It indicates the dysfunction of dorsal columns.

In Romberg's test, a patient is asked to stand with the feet as close together as possible. The patient is then observed with his or her eyes closed. An abnormal result consists of swaying or other evidence of instability.

Damage in which brain region is most likely to result in impaired social judgment?

Orbitofrontal area.

What are the features of giant-cell arteritis?

In a typical case of giant-cell arteritis, an elderly patient reports very severe headache associated at times with periods of monocular visual loss. The patient also has aches in various joints and some stiffness in the morning. Another typical manifestation is jaw pain.

Laboratory finding: Increased erythrocyte sedimentation rate.

Diagnostic test: Temporal artery biopsy.

Treatment: High-dose steroids.

What are the pros and cons of CT and MRI of the head?

CT: Economical, more available, the diagnostic procedure of choice for acute hemorrhage or acute trauma, suitable for pacemaker bearers.

MRI: Better differentiation of white from gray matter, better identification of white-matter lesions, better detection of posterior fossa and brain-stem pathology, suitable for patients for whom radiation exposure is contraindicated (e.g., during pregnancy).

What does a go-no go test evaluate?

Frontal–subcortical-system tasks.

In the go-no go test, the patient taps the underside of a table twice when the examiner taps the underside of the table once; when the examiner taps twice, the patient makes no response.

What is diabetic mononeuropathy simplex?

A condition likely to stem from the involvement of a cranial nerve. The likelihood of involvement follows the order: Oculomotor (III), abducens (VI), and trochlear (IV) nerve.

The presentation involves a diabetic patient who has a periorbital headache of sudden onset on the right and diplopia of new onset. Examination shows right eyelid ptosis and an inability to adduct or elevate the right eye. The pupils react normally to light directly and consensually. There is no pallor of the optic disk.

What is anosognosia?

A body image disorder caused by a parietal lobe lesion and which takes the form of unilateral neglect. The patient tends not to use the contralateral limbs, may deny that there is anything wrong with these limbs, and may even fail to recognize the contralateral limbs.

What are the lesion locations and clinic characteristics of aphasia?

Frontal lobe:

Broca's aphasia (expressive, nonfluent aphasia): Good comprehension but poor repetition and fluency. Paucity of speech; halting, agrammatic speech;

telegraphic speech. Associated with hemiparesis.

Posterior temporal lobe:

Wernickes's aphasia (receptive, fluent aphasia): Good speech fluency but poor comprehension and poor repetition. Intact grammar, neologisms, paraphasias, word salad, and nonsensical speech. Associated with a reduction in the visual field.

Arcuate fasciculus:

Conduction aphasia: Good speech comprehension and fluency but poor repetition.

What is the most consistent biochemical finding in Alzheimer's disease?

A deficiency in choline acetyltransferase.

What are the common findings in normal-pressure hydrocephalus?

The triad of ataxia, urinary incontinence, and dementia. Enlarged ventricles can be seen by CT or MRI.

Treatment: Surgical bypass shunting.

What are the clinical manifestations of an embolic stroke in left angular gyrus?

The patient has fluent speech and excellent comprehension but is unable to name fingers and body parts or to determine right or left orientation, unable to write down thoughts and take notes but has good reading comprehension, and unable to do calculations.

What is the function of the suprachiasmatic nucleus?

The organization of behavioral and physiologic circadian rhythm.

What is hemiballismus?

A unilateral chorea that is especially violent because the proximal muscles of the limbs are involved.

This condition is classically attributed to vascular disease in the contralateral subthalamic nucleus.

Recent data suggest that lesions located in the caudate or other basal ganglia are more likely to be associated with hemiballismus than are lesions in other areas. The possible causes of hemiballismus include toxoplasmosis secondary to human immunodeficiency virus infection, and vasculitis.

Hemiballismus commonly resolves spontaneously within weeks. Dopamine-blocking agents may suppress the abnormal movements in this condition.

What is idiopathic Bell's palsy?

Facial weakness (inability to close the eye, drooping of the face) of the lower-motor-neuron type, without evidence of aural or more widespread neurologic disease. It is preceded by pain about the ear, and may be associated with <u>impairment of taste</u> or lacrimation, or with <u>hyperacusis</u> (sensitivity to <u>loud, low-frequency sounds</u>).

What is syringomyelia?

Cavitation of the spinal cord, commonly occurring in the cervical region.

Typically, there is a dissociated sensory loss at the level of the lesion: Pinprick and temperature appreciation are impaired, but light touch and vibration sensation are preserved.

Weakness and wasting of muscles occur at the level of the lesion, and reflexes are absent.

What is the major location of subacute combined degeneration of the spinal cord in pernicious anemia?

Posterior and lateral funiculi.

What are the manifestations of optic-nerve pathology?

Impairment of visual acuity in one eye. Direct and consensual responses to light are weak on the diseased side but not on the other side.

What is the clinical presentation of Klüver–Bucy syndrome?

Emotional placidity and compulsive oral behavior.

The site of pathology is amygdaloid nucleus.

What are the characteristics of cluster headache?

Quality of pain: Brief, very severe (excruciating, sharp stabbing), nonthrobbing, unilateral headache that recurs on the same side, retro-orbitally and/or in the nostril.

Time: Nighttime occurrence, awakening the patient from sleep; may recur in the day. Duration from 10 minutes to 2 hours.

Other symptoms: Ipsilateral lacrimation (tearing), conjunctival injection, nasal stuffiness, and Horner's syndrome.

Frequently occurs in men; mean age at onset is 25 years.

What is the neuropathologic hallmark of Marchiafava–Bignami disease?

Atrophy and demyelination of the corpus callosum.

Marchiafava–Bignami disease occurs most often in malnourished alcoholics.

The clinical features are dementia, spasticity, dysarthria, and gait disturbance.

What are major pathologic features of idiopathic Parkisonism?

Loss of pigmentation and cells in the substantia nigra.

Cell loss in the globus pallidus and putamen.

Presence of <u>eosinophilic intraneural inclusion granules (Lewy bodies)</u> in the basal ganglia, brainstem, spinal cord, and sympathetic ganglia.

Lewy bodies may appear in many forms of Parkinsonism, but not in postencephalitic Parkinsonism.

What clinical feature can differentiate complex partial seizures from simple partial seizures?

Complex partial seizures are marked by an altered responsiveness to outside stimuli without loss of consciousness, whereas in simple partial seizures there is no change in responsiveness to outside stimuli.

What are the characteristics of neurosyphilis?

<u>Dementia</u> and other psychiatric presentations.

CT shows <u>generalized atrophy.</u>

The CSF contains <u>lymphocytes and protein. Gamma globulin</u> is elevated.

What is the most important condition to be considered in a senile patient with headaches and pain in the jaw muscles when chewing?

Temporal arteritis.

What are the clinical features of diabetic neuropathy?

1. Sensory deficits, including <u>pain</u> and <u>paresthesia.</u>
2. Motor deficits, presenting as muscle weakness and <u>atrophy.</u>
3. Autonomic neuropathy, presenting as <u>postural hypotension,</u> neurogenic bladder, and incontinence.

Sample Questions

1. A 70-year-old male patient presents with progressive dementia. A magnetic resonance imaging (MRI) scan shows multiple areas of increased T2-weighted density in the periventricular area. What is the most likely diagnosis?

A. Pseudotumor cerebri.
B. Normal-pressure hydrocephalus.
C. Multi-infarct dementia.
D. Pick's disease.
E. Metastatic carcinoma.

The answer is C.

The MRI finding is pathognomonic for multi-infarct dementia.

Pseudotumor cerebri: MRI shows small ventricles.

Normal-pressure hydrocephalus: MRI shows enlarged lateral ventricles.

Pick's disease: MRI shows frontal- and temporal-lobe atrophy.

Metastatic carcinoma: MRI shows multiple coin-like lesions.

2. Neuroleptic malignant syndrome (NMS) commonly presents with each of the following EXCEPT:

A. Elevated creatine kinase.
B. Rigidity and tremor.
C. Leukopenia.
D. Labile blood pressure.
E. Fever.

The answer is C.

NMS is usually associated with leukocytosis, not leukopenia.

3. Focal dystonia (blepharospasm, oromandibular dystonia, spasmodic torticollis, writer's cramp, etc.) can be effectively treated with:

A. Haloperidol.
B. Reserpine.
C. Surgical denervation.
D. Botulinum toxin.
E. Baclofen.

The answer is D.

Haloperidol, an antipsychotic agent, can be used in the treatment of Gilles de la Tourette's syndrome.

Baclofen is a centrally acting muscle relaxant and can be used in the treatment of trigeminal neuralgia and other painful spasms. It is not an effective treatment for focal dystonia.

Reserpine and surgical denervation are not usually used in treating focal dystonia.

4. A 25-year-old male complains of recurrent severe headache. He states that his headache usually occurs in the early morning. Sometimes he was awakened by headache. The pain lasts from 30 to 60 minutes. It is excruciating and stabbing. The pain begins at his left nostril, and this is followed by severe retro-orbital pain. It is accompanied by tearing and nasal stuffiness on the left side of the face. The patient's mother, who has witnessed his episodes, has noted injection of his left eye and swelling of the left side of his face during the headache. The most likely diagnosis is:

A. Giant-cell arteritis.
B. Trigeminal neuralgia.
C. Migraine.
D. Cluster headache.
E. Glaucoma.

The answer is D.

Giant-cell arteritis is seen primarily in the elderly. The onset is abrupt or insidious over a period of weeks. Typical symptoms include unilateral headache involving the jaw, tongue, and temporal region, and visual disturbances. Eye injection and facial swelling are not associated with this condition.

Trigeminal neuralgia produces severe pain in the distribution of one or more of the divisions of the trigeminal nerve, most commonly the second or third division. Symptoms rarely present at night. The pain may be elicited by tickle or touch. The pain usually occurs in bursts lasting several seconds, which are followed by a refractory period.

Migraine is a paroxysmal headache lasting for hours to days, with or without an aura. The pain is usually unilateral, throbbing, and intensified by movement. Sleep may abort the pain.

Glaucoma presents with a dull ache in or around one eye, with mildly blurred vision and halos around lights. Symptoms occur when watching television or reading in a dark room.

5. All of the following occur in normal pressure hydrocephalus EXCEPT:

A. Gait disturbance (ataxia).
B. Enlarged ventricles.
C. Urinary incontinence.
D. Dementia.
E. Positive Romberg's sign.

The answer is E.

A positive Romberg's sign usually presents in spinal conditions.

6. A left-handed female had a recent cerebral vascular accident. She is able to comprehend and follow commands. However, she is unable to speak with correct grammar, and cannot repeat other people's words. Her speech is nonfluent and telegraphic. All of the following are correct EXCEPT:

A. This patient most likely also has a visual-field reduction.
B. This is a case of Broca's aphasia.
C. The cerebral lesion involves the left frontal lobe.
D. The patient most likely also has right hemiparesis.
E. The patient's type of aphasia is also known as expressive aphasia.

The answer is A.

A visual-field reduction is a symptom associated with disturbance in the optic tract, optic chiasm, or optic nerve, and not with a cortical disturbance. Broca's area is not associated with visual function.

In the majority (80%) of left-handed people, the left cerebrum is the dominant side.

7. The following are contraindicated for concomitant use with monamine oxidase inhibitors (MAOIs) EXCEPT:

A. Meperidine.
B. Aged cheese.
C. Phentolamine.   *Agonist used for*
D. Phenylephrine.   *MAOI - HTN crisis*
E. Fluoxetine.

The answer is C.

Phentolamine is an α-adrenergic antagonist that may be used to treat MAOI-related hypertensive crises.

8. Which of the following is NOT a characteristic feature of complex partial seizures?

A. A commonly associated symptom is an epigastric sensation.
B. Affect is usually flattened.
C. Consciousness is impaired but not lost.
D. Olfactory hallucination and déjà vu may appear.
E. The majority of patients present with automatism.

The answer is B.

Complex partial seizures are associated with intensified affect.

9. A 30-year-old woman complains of severe headaches and episodes of brief loss of vision. She states that she has been depressed and has gained 50 pounds in the past 12 months. A neurologic examination yields insignificant findings except for bilateral papilledema. An MRI scan of the brain shows small ventricles. Lumber puncture reveals elevated cerebrospinal fluid (CSF) pressure. What is the most likely diagnosis?

A. Pseudotumor cerebri.
B. Normal-pressure hydrocephalus.
C. Major depressive disorder (MDD).
D. Bacterial meningitis.
E. Metastatic carcinoma.

The answer is A.

Normal-pressure hydrocephalus: MRI shows enlarged lateral ventricles. CSF pressure is not elevated.

MDD: No significant neurologic effect.

Meningitis: Usually no change in the MRI.

Metastatic carcinoma: Typical MRI finding is multiple coin-like lesions.

10. A 35-year-old female patient suffers from progressive dementia and involuntary dance-like movements. She has a positive family history of these same manifestations. Genetic study reports an expansion of CAG trinucleotide repeat sequences at chromosome 4p16.3. Which of the following agents is the best treatment for the patient's abnormal involuntary movements?

A. Benztropine.
B. Haloperidol.
C. L-Dihydroxyphenylalanine (L-DOPA).
D. Stereotactic thalamotomy.
E. Lorazepam.

The answer is B.

This is a typical case of Huntington's disease. Haloperidol is the treatment of choice.

Benztropine is a treatment for drug-induced parkinsonism.

L-DOPA is a treatment for Parkinson's disease.

Stereotactic thalamotomy is a treatment for intractable seizure.

Lorazepam is used in a variety of disorders. Its intravenous (IV) form is particularly useful for aborting seizure. It is not effective for Huntington's disease.

11. In older populations, drug metabolism is changed by the following factor(s):

A. Decrease in body fat.
B. Increased perfusion of the liver.
C. Increased plasma-binding proteins.
D. Increased renal clearance.
E. Decreased hepatic metabolism.

The answer is E.

The metabolic change in elderly persons is in the opposite direction from all of the listed statements except E.

12. A 49-year-old male patient experiences progressive weakness for several months. He also complains of muscle twitching, cramps, easy fatigability, and stiffness in his arms and legs. Physical examination shows atrophy of the intrinsic muscles, and the reflexes are brisk. There are no sensory findings. Electrophysiologic study shows widespread fasciculations, fibrillation, and positive sharp waves. The history and results of examinations strongly suggest which of the following diagnoses?

A. Multiple sclerosis.
B. Fascioscapulohumeral muscular dystrophy.
C. Amyotrophic lateral sclerosis.
D. Chronic fatigue.
E. Myasthenia gravis.

The answer is C.

Multiple sclerosis: Involves different parts of the central nervous system (CNS). Symptoms are often transient, disappearing after a few days or weeks. They may include changes in vision and disturbances in bladder function. Sensory deficits may appear. Diagnosis is based on the clinical picture, CSF findings (oligoclonal bands), MRI, and other tests.

Fascioscapulohumeral muscular dystrophy: Rearrangement of a homeobox gene on the long arm of chromosome 4. Onset in adolescence. Weakness is confined to the face, neck, and shoulder.

Chronic fatigue syndrome should not have any neurologic signs.

Myasthenia gravis: Impaired neuromuscular transmission. Most cases involve extraocular muscles. Sustained activity of affected muscles leads to temporarily increased weakness. Sensation is normal. No reflex changes. Electrophysiological testing shows decremental responses of muscle to repetitive supramaximal stimulation of the muscle motor nerve, but normal findings are aslo possible.

13. A 39-year-old woman experiences progressive weakness of her arms and legs over a period of several days. Physical examination reveals symmetric weakness and absence of deep tendon reflexes. CSF testing shows an elevated protein with 6 lymphocytes/mm³. Nerve-conduction study reports show a slow conduction velocity, prolonged distal motor latency, and conduction block. What is the most likely diagnosis?

A. Polymyositis.
B. Guillain-Barré syndrome
C. Myasthenia gravis.
D. Normal pressure hydrocephalus.
E. Amyotrophic lateral sclerosis.

The answer is B.

Polymyositis: Rare in developed countries. Weakness is accompanied by myalgia and signs of meningeal irritation, and is asymmetric in distribution. Diagnosis is based on the isolation of the virus from the stool and/or nasopharyngeal secretions, and less commonly from the CSF.

Myasthenia gravis: Impaired neuromuscular transmission. Most cases involve extraocular muscles. Sustained activity of affected muscles leads to temporarily increased weakness. Sensation is normal. No changes in reflexes. Electrophysiologic testing shows decremental responses of muscle to repetitive supramaximal stimulation of the muscle motor nerve, but normal findings are also possible.

Normal-pressure hydrocephalus: MRI shows enlarged lateral ventricles. No elevated CSF pressure. No change in nerve conduction.

Amyotrophic lateral sclerosis: Mixed upper- and lower-motor-neuron deficit. No change in nerve conduction. No abnormalities in CSF tests.

14. The following are effective treatments for obsessive-compulsive disorder EXCEPT:

A. Paroxetine 50 mg per day.
B. Clomipramine 250 mg per day.
C. Phenelzine 15 mg t.i.d.
D. Fluoxetine 20 mg per day.
E. Fluvoxamine 150 mg b.i.d.

The answer is D.

The treatment of obsessive-compulsive disorder requires a high-dose antidepressant with a serotonergic effect.

15. Neurologic examination of a 72-year-old man reveals postural instability and a tendency to accelerate involuntarily with small steps. The patient walks with rigid, shuffling steps and a narrow base. There is a tendency to lean forward to accelerate the speed of walking. The clinical presentation is typical for:

A. Sensory ataxia.
B. Alcoholic cerebellar degeneration.
C. Normal aging.
D. Huntington's chorea.
E. Parkinson's disease.

The answer is E.

Sensory ataxia: A syndrome that may be caused by polyneuropathy and myelopathy. Impaired proprioceptive sensation exists at all the levels of the sensory pathway. Defective joint position, a positive Romberg's sign, and a slapping or steppage gait are typical symptoms of sensory ataxia.

Alcoholic cerebellar degeneration: Usually restricted to the superior vermis. Gait ataxia, distal sensory deficits in the feet, and absent ankle reflexes are common symptoms.

Normal aging may be associated with general weakness and slowness, but not with the typical parkinsonian symptoms described above.

Huntington's chorea: Typical onset is between 30 and 50 years of age. The condition terminates fatally 10 to 20 years after clinical onset. Chorea is manifested as dancelike gross movements. In the early stage of the disease, fidgeting or restlessness may appear. Diagnosis is based on genetic testing, which shows expanded CAG trinucleotide repeat sequences in the short arm of chromosome 4.

16. Indications for psychostimulants are all of the following EXCEPT:

A. ADHD.
B. Personality disorders.
C. Narcolepsy.
D. Exogenous obesity.
E. Depression in elderly and medically ill patients.

The answer is B.

Psychostimulants should not be used in personality disorders or for patients with a history of substance abuse.

17. A 43-year-old woman complains of recurrent episodes of severe vertigo with nausea and vomiting. The symptoms usually occur with a change in head position, and are most severe in the lateral decubitus position with the left ear facing down. Neurologic examination reveals left-sided nystagmus before the occurrence of symptoms when the patient is moved from a sitting to a recumbent position. Upon repeated positional testing, the patient's symptoms are found to become less severe. Her hearing is normal. Neurologic examination is otherwise insignificant. The most likely diagnosis is:

A. Ménière's disease.
B. Basilar artery insufficiency.
C. Orthostatic hypotension.
D. Cerebellar infarct.
E. Benign positional vertigo.

The answer is E.

Ménière's disease: Vertigo is not associated with changes in head position. Hearing deteriorates in Ménière's disease.

Basilar artery insufficiency: Although auditory nerve is supplied by a branch of the basilar artery, basilar artery insufficiency usually involves many other structures, and always involves the dorsal portion of the pons. It causes abducens nerve palsy, impaired horizontal eye movements, and vertical nystagmus. Hemiplegia or quadriplegia is usually present, and coma is common.

Orthostatic hypotension: Dizziness, lightheadedness, but no vertigo.

Cerebellar infarct: Coma of acute onset, and rapid deterioration that leads to death.

18. Electroconvulsive therapy (ECT) is likely to be effective for the following conditions EXCEPT:

A. Catatonia.
B. Delirium.
C. Acute mania.
D. Severe depression.
E. Somatization disorder.

The answer is E.

ECT is not effective in somatization disorder, personality disorders, or anxiety disorders.

19. A 40-year-old woman complains of persistent numbness on the palmar surface of her right hand, and of pain in her right arm. Her symptoms are more severe in the morning. Neurologic examination reveals a sensory deficit in the right thumb, index, and middle fingers, as well as on the lateral half of the ring finger. The patient has weakness in abducting the thumb. Laboratory tests reveal an elevated level of thyroid stimulating hormone. Which of the following is the most likely diagnosis?

A. Ulnar nerve entrapment.
B. Radial nerve compression.
C. Carpal tunnel syndrome.
D. Radial fracture.
E. Atherosclerosis.

The answer is C.

Ulnar nerve entrapment impairs adduction of the little finger. There is a sensory deficit on the palmar surface and back of the little finger and on the lateral side of the ring finger.

Radial nerve compression: Difficulty in adducting (not abducting) the thumb. There is a sensory deficit on the back of the hand between the thumb and index finger.

Radial fracture: May be associated with radial nerve damage.

Atherosclerosis: No typical distribution of deficits as described in this case.

20. Many drugs may change the serum lithium level. In the following list, the drug that may decrease the serum lithium level is:

A. Nonsteroidal anti-inflammatory drug.
B. Ibuprofen.
C. Indomethacin.
D. Theophylline.
E. Spironolactone.

The answer is D.

Theophylline is the only one of the drugs listed that may decrease the serum lithium level. All of the remaining drugs may increase serum lithium levels.

21. Which of the following medicines is associated with the development of ataxia, gingival hyperplasia, hirsutism, agranulocytosis, and coarse facial features?

A. Phenytoin.
B. Carbamazepine.
C. Valproic acid.
D. Topiramate.
E. Oxcarbazepine.

The answer is A.

Ataxia, although it has a neurologic definition, may be clinically difficult to differentiate from many forms of gait unsteadiness, and therefore is too general a term to point to a specific drug.

Gingival hyperplasia is a specific reaction to phenytoin. Another anticonvulsant that may have similar reaction is ethosuximide.

Many drugs may promote extra hair growth. Phenytoin is a well-known such drug. Valproic acid may cause hair loss. Carbamazepine and topiramate are not associated with hirsutism.

Hirsutism in oxcarbazepine users is rare.

Agranulocytosis is associated with many drugs. Of the drugs listed, only topiramate is not associated with bone-marrow suppression.

22. A 9-year-old boy is observed to have several episodes of brief "out-of-mind" spells. His family notices that in such spells he suddenly stops his activities, blinks his eyes, and turns his head to the left. Each spell lasts a couple of seconds. The boy never falls during these spells, and recovers completely to a normal state. What is the appropriate treatment for this boy?

A. Carbamazepine.
B. Valproic acid.
C. Lamotrigine.
D. Gabapentin.
E. Phenytoin.

The answer is B.

This boy suffers from absence seizures, also known as petit mal seizures. Treatment consists of ethosuximide (Zarontin) and valproic acid.

23. In order to obtain therapeutic effect from ECT, which of the following is required?

A. Loss of consciousness.
B. Electrical stimulation of the left hemisphere.
C. Bilateral spread of convulsion.
D. Induction of amnesia.
E. Anesthesia.

The answer is C.

Bilateral convulsion is the only one of the foregoing conditions in which there is consistent evidence of a therapeutic effect of ECT.

24. All of the following are choices of pharmacologic treatment in attention-deficit/hyperactivity disorder (AD/HD) EXCEPT:

A. Methylphenidate.
B. Bupropion.
C. Clonidine.
D. Propranolol.
E. Pemoline.

The answer is D.

Choices for treatment of AD/HD are stimulants, antidepressants, and clonidine.

25. What is the treatment of choice for lithium-induced polyuria and polydipsia?

A. Reduce fluid intake.
B. Amiloride.
C. Propranolol.
D. Mannitol.
E. Furosemide.

The answer is B.

Lithium inhibits free-water resorption at the collecting tubule. Amiloride is a potassium-sparing diuretic that inhibits sodium resorption at the distal convoluted tubule. Amiloride can reduce the symptoms of polyuria and polydipsia.

Reducing fluid intake, mannitol, and furosemide worsen the symptoms of lithium-induced polyuria and polydipsia. Propranolol is useful in treating lithium-induced tremor, not polyuria/polydipsia.

26. What is the most common side effect of clozapine?

A. Seizure.
B. Agranulocytosis.
C. Hypotension.
D. Sedation.
E. Increased prolactin level.

The answer is D.

Seizure and agranulocytosis are both rare but severe, and hence notorious, adverse reactions to clozapine. Clozapine may cause hypotension, but the most common side effect is sedation. Clozapine has minimal effect on serum prolactin levels, which is one of the features that make it the "gold standard" of atypical antipsychotic agents.

27. Which of the following is not a symptom of serotonin syndrome?

A. Jitteriness and tremor.
B. Hypotension.
C. Hypotonicity.
D. Diaphoresis.
E. Hypertension.

The answer is C.

Hypertonicity may appear in serotonin syndrome.

Autonomic instability is one of the key features of serotonin syndrome. It may present with either hypo- or hypertension.

28. Mirtazapine is a unique antidepressant that blocks the following receptors EXCEPT:

A. Type-1 histamine receptor (H1).
B. α₂-Adrenergic receptor (α₂).
C. Type-1 serotonin receptor (5HT1).
D. Type-2 serotonin receptor (5HT2).
E. Type-3 serotonin receptor (5HT3).

The answer is C.

Mirtazapine blocks central α_2-adrenergic receptors and increases serotonergic tone. It blocks 5HT2 and 5HT3 receptors, reducing anxiety and gastrointestinal (GI) reactivity, and enhances serotonergic binding to 5HT1A and 5HT1C receptors. Mirtazapine also blocks H1 receptors, which gives mirtazapine its sedative effect.

29. Bupropion is contraindicated in patients with:

A. Myocardial infarction.
B. Alcohol dependence.
C. Obesity.
D. Sexual dysfunction.
E. Eating disorder.

The answer is E.

Another important contraindication to bupropion is seizure disorder.

Bupropion is not contraindicated in cardiac conditions or in alcohol/drug dependence. Bupropion may reduce sexual dysfunction induced by serotonin-specific reuptake inhibitors (SSRIs), and even improves sexual function in some cases. One of the side effects of bupropion is weight loss.

30. The reaction to anticipated death, according to Elizabeth Kubler-Ross, includes which of the following orders of stages:

A. Denial, anger, bargaining, depression, and acceptance.
B. Denial, shock, anger, bargaining, and acceptance.
C. Denial, depression, bargaining, anger, acceptance.
D. Shock, anger, bargaining, acceptance, and gratefulness.
E. Denial, rumination, bargaining, anger, acceptance.

The answer is A.

1. Shock and denial.
2. Anger.
3. Bargaining.
4. Depression.
5. Acceptance.

31. The characteristic features of Rett's disorder are the following EXCEPT:

A. Deceleration of head growth beginning in early childhood.
B. Macro-orchidism.
C. Loss of previously acquired purposeful hand skills.
D. Loss of social engagement.
E. Severely impaired language development.

The answer is B.

Macro-orchidism is a feature of Fragile X syndrome, not of Rett's disorder.

32. According to Erik Erikson, the developmental crisis most typical of normal teenagers involves:

A. Initiative versus guilt.
B. Intimacy versus isolation.
C. Ego integrity versus despair.
D. Identity versus role confusion.
E. Autonomy versus shame and doubt.

The answer is D.

Basic trust versus mistrust: Age 0 to 1 year.

Autonomy versus shame and doubt: Age 1 to 3 years.

Initiative versus guilt: Age 3 to 6 years.

Industry versus inferiority: Age 6 to 12 years.

Identity versus role confusion: Age 12 to 20 years.

Intimacy versus isolation: Age 20 to 40 years.

Generativity versus stagnation: Age 40 to 65 years.

Ego integrity versus despair: Age 65 years and older.

33. Orthostatic hypotension and priapism are associated with which of the following effects?

A. α_1-Adrenergic receptor stimulation.
B. α_1-Adrenergic receptor blockade.
C. α_2-Adrenergic receptor stimulation.
D. α_2-Adrenergic receptor blockade.
E. Muscarinic cholinergic receptor blockade.

The answer is B.

α_1-Adrenergic receptor stimulation may cause vascular contraction, and result in elevation of blood pressure.

α_2-Adrenergic receptor is a presynaptic receptor. Stimulation of α_2-adrenergic receptors may cause decreased release of norepinephrine and serotonin (e.g., as with clonidine). Blockade of α_2-adrenergic receptors increases the release of norepinephrine and serotonin (e.g., as with mirtazapine).

An anticholinergic effect may cause dizziness and drowsiness, which is similar to what occurs with α_1-adrenergic receptor blockade. However, cholinergic receptors do not have a direct effect on vascular activity.

34. Adverse effects of lithium include the following EXCEPT:

A. Tremor.
B. Nephrogenic diabetes insipidus.
C. Weight gain.
D. Hypothyroidism.
E. Exacerbation of narrow-angle glaucoma.

The answer is E.

An anticholinergic effect is associated with exacerbation of narrow-angle glaucoma. Lithium does not have an anticholinergic effect.

35. The following are associated with the effect of venlafaxine, EXCEPT:

A. Blockade of serotonin reuptake.
B. Blockade of norepinephrine reuptake.
C. Blockade of dopamine reuptake.
D. Possibly elevated systolic but not diastolic blood pressure.
E. No significant inhibition of cytochrome P450.

The answer is D.

Venlafaxine mainly causes elevated diastolic blood pressure.

36. The "learned helplessness" animal model is proposed for the research of which of the following psychiatric illnesses?

A. Schizophrenia.
B. Anxiety.
C. Depression.
D. Mania.
E. Aggression.

The answer is C.

"Learned helplessness" is one of the many animal models for the study of depression. Others include pharmacologic models (e.g., the reserpine syndrome model); separation models (maternal separation or peer separation); and chronic stress models, as well as others.

Drug-related (amphetamine, phencyclidine, and hallucinogen) animal models and sensorimotor-gating models of schizophrenia are commonly applied to schizophrenia research.

Operant conditioning paradigms are usually used to establish animal models for the study of anxiety.

For mania and aggression, there is so far no commonly used animal model.

37. What method of producing a stimulus could make an experimental animal most resistant to extinction?

A. A fixed-interval schedule
B. A fixed-ratio schedule.
C. A variable-ratio schedule.
D. Positive reinforcement.

The answer is C.

The most difficult way to extinguish a stimulus is to produce it on a variable-ratio schedule, or in an intermittent, relatively unpredictable fashion. The fixed-ratio schedule causes habituation but not resistance to extinction. Positive reinforcement is necessary for creating resistance to extinction, but the means of delivery of the stimulus is more important. Consider a mediocre researcher who occasionally gets a paper published and gets low level grants once every few years. It is very hard for such a person to give up his or her effort because reinforcement provided is on a variable-ratio schedule!

38. A 2-year-old boy has strong attachment to his parents. What will be his reaction when he sees his parents return to the room in which he is present after a brief separation from him?

A. Continued play.
B. Brief contact followed by continued play.
C. Intense anger.
D. Sustained contact and cessation of play.
E. Avoidance of the parents.

The answer is B.

Based on Mary Ainsworth's study, more than 60% of children develop secure attachments by the age of 24 months. Attachment is the bonding that develops between a child and its primary caregiver. Children usually consider their primary caregiver as the symbol of security and resources available to them.

In this case, the typical reaction of the child is brief contact followed by continued play.

39. Applying positive and negative stimuli to alter the frequency of behavior is called:

A. Classical conditioning.
B. Operant conditioning.
C. Partial reinforcement.
D. Respondent learning.
E. Higher-order conditioning.

The answer is B.

Also known as instrumental conditioning, operant conditioning is a form of learning in which behavioral frequency is altered through the application of positive and negative consequences. B.F. Skinner developed the theory of operant conditioning. As an example of such conditioning, a dog might receive food only when it correctly responds by pressing a lever. Food is the reinforcing stimulus and the lever is the operant.

Classical conditioning, developed by Ivan Pavlov, results from the repeated pairing of a neutral (conditioned) stimulus with one that evokes a response (unconditioned stimulus), such that the neutral stimulus eventually comes to evoke the response. This is also called respondent learning. The establishing of a new conditioned stimulus through coupling with an established stimulus is called higher-order conditioning.

Partial reinforcement means that reinforcement of a particular behavior occurs intermittently. This makes the behavior highly resistant to extinction.

40. Based on Sigmund Freud's theory, what does a 4-year-old boy fear?

A. Castration by his father.
B. Aggression toward his mother.
C. Death of his father.
D. Identification with his father.

The answer is A.

This boy is in his phallic phase and could have castration anxiety. Another possible presentation could be an Oedipus complex.

The other items in the questions are confusing.

Sigmund Freud's stages of psychosexual development are:

1. Oral (birth to 18 months).
2. Anal (1 to 3 years).
3. Phallic (oedipal, 3 to 5 years).
4. Latency (5 to 12 years).
5. Genital (12 years to adulthood).

41. What is the Wisconsin Card Sorting Test indicated to evaluate?

A. Malingering.
B. Visual–spatial memory.
C. Attention.
D. Executive functions.

The answer is D.

In the Wisconsin Card Sorting Test (WCST), the test-taker is required to match his response cards to the stimulus card by following certain rules (such as color, form, and number). The rules change without notification of the test-taker, but the correct response is learned by feedback. The test-taker needs to recognize the current rules and follow them in the card-playing process. In this way, the test-taker's executive function is examined.

The best test for detecting malingering is the clinical interview. The neuropsychologic test that helps in this regard is the Minnesota Multiphasic Personality Inventory (MMPI).

Visual–spatial memory is tested with the Rey–Osterreith Complex Figure test or Draw-a-Clock Face test.

Attention and concentration are tested with the Digit Span test of the Wechsler Adult Intelligence Scale-III (WAIS–III) or with the Trail-Making test Parts A and B.

42. All of the following are projective tests EXCEPT:

A. Rorschach Test.
B. Thematic Apperception Test.
C. Sentence Completion Test.
D. MMPI.

E. Draw-a-person test.

The answer is D.

The MMPI is not a projective test.

The remaining projective tests can detect subtle psychotic thought processes and bizarre ideation.

43. What does the comprehension subtest of the WAIS measure?

A. Attention and concentration.
B. Receptive and expressive language.
C. Ability to abstract.
D. Memory function.

The answer is C.

In WAIS-III:

The Comprehension subtest measures executive functions and abstract thinking.

The Mental Control subtest of the Wechsler Memory Scale-III (WMS-III) and WAIS-III Digit Span test measure attention and concentration.

The Verbal Intelligence Quotient (IQ) subtest measures receptive and expressive language function.

The WMS-III measures memory function.

WAIS-III itself measures adult (16 to 89 years) general intelligence. The Wechsler Preschool and Primary Scale of Intelligence is for children aged 4 to 6 years. The Wechsler Intelligence Scale for Children-III is for children aged 5 to 16 years. Three major IQ test-score components are: Full-scale IQ, Verbal IQ, and Performance IQ.

44. Researchers conduct a study by following a group of subjects chosen from a well-defined population over a period of time. This type of study is a:

A. **Cohort study.**
B. **Cross-sectional study.**
C. **Case-control study.**
D. **Case-history study.**
E. **Retrospective study.**

The answer is A.

Cohort study (also known as follow up study): A group of individuals (cohort) is defined on the basis of the presence or absence of exposure to a suspected risk factor for a disease, and is followed for an extended period. A cohort study is a form of prospective study.

Case–control study: Subjects are selected on the basis of whether they do or do not have a particular disease being studied.

45. What is the term for the relative frequency of a condition in a population as measured at a particular point in time?

A. **Sensitivity.**
B. **Specificity.**
C. **Incidence.**
D. **Prevalence.**

The answer is D.

Prevalence is the proportion of individuals with <u>existing disease</u> at a point in time (point prevalence) or during a period of time (period prevalence). It refers to all persons who are diseased within a given population.

Incidence is the proportion of individuals developing <u>new disease</u> during a period of time.

It refers only to new cases of disease.

Sensitivity measures the ability of a test to identify true-positive cases of disease. Specificity measures the ability of a test to identify true-negative cases of the disease.

46. You encourage your patient to stop smoking so as to reduce the patient's risk of getting lung cancer. Which type of prevention is this?

A. Primary prevention.
B. Secondary prevention.
C. Tertiary prevention.
D. Not prevention, just a suggestion.

The answer is A.

Primary prevention: To prevent the onset of a disease and thereby reduce its incidence by eliminating the causative agents, reducing risk factors, enhancing host resistance, and interfering with disease transmission.

Secondary prevention: Early identification and prompt treatment of an illness, with the goal of reducing the prevalence of the condition by reducing its duration.

Tertiary prevention: Reducing the prevalence of residual defects and disabilities caused by an illness. This enables persons with chronic mental illnesses to reach the highest feasible level of function.

47. You recommend vocational therapy to your schizophrenia patients after they have been stable for some period of time. Which type of prevention is this?

A. Primary prevention.
B. Secondary prevention.
C. Tertiary prevention.
D. Not prevention, just a recommendation.

The answer is C.

Please do not make mistake on this topic. Read the above answer for reference.

48. A social worker helps psychiatric patients obtain the services already available from the community. Which kind of service model is this?

A. Assertive community treatment.
B. Traditional social work.
C. Both.
D. Neither.

The answer is B.

Assertive community treatment: Active outreach to patients.

Traditional social work: Helps patients connect to existing services.

49. What is the most common cause of death among male African–American youths?

A. Suicide.
B. Homicide.
C. Traffic accident.
D. Substance abuse.

The answer is B.

Homicide is the most common cause of death among young African–American males.

50. The major inhibitory neurotransmitter in the central nervous system (CNS) is:

A. Glutamate.
B. γ-Aminobutyric acid (GABA).
C. Dopamine.
D. Serotonin.

The answer is B.

GABA is the major inhibitory neurotransmitter in the CNS. Glycine is the major inhibitory neurotransmitter in the brain stem and peripheral nervous system (PNS). Glutamate is the major excitatory neurotransmitter in the CNS and PNS. Both dopamine and serotonin are regulatory neurotransmitters.

51. The cell bodies of which type of neuron are located in the Ventral Tegmental Area (VTA)?

A. Dopaminergic.
B. Serotonergic.
C. Noradrenergic.
D. GABAergic.

The answer is A.

1. Dopaminergic: Three locations.
   A. Substantia nigra (<u>nigrostriatal pathway,</u> associated with extrapyramidal syndromes [EPS]).
   B. VTA, mesolimbic-mesocortical pathway associated with antipsychotic effects, and reward system.
   C. Hypothalamus, including the arcuate and periventricular nuclei (tuberoinfundibular pathway, associated with prolactin regulation).
2. Serotoninergic:
   A. <u>Raphe nuclei</u> (upper pons and midbrain).
   B. Caudal locus coeruleus (to a lesser extent).
3. Noradrenergic: <u>Locus coeuleus</u> (pons).
4. GABAergic: GABAergic neurons are small interneurons prevalent throughout the CNS.

52. Of which hormone has dopamine been shown to inhibit the release?

A. **Thyroid-stimulating hormone.**
B. **Follicle-stimulating hormone.**
C. **Luteinizing hormone.**
D. **Antidiuretic hormone.**
E. **Prolactin.**

The answer is E.

Dopamine inhibits the release of prolactin through the tuberoinfundibular pathway.

53. Based on biologic study, the level in CSF of which of the following factors is inversely related to aggressive behavior?

A. Glutamate.
B. Histamine.
C. Neuropeptide Y.
D. 5-Hydroxyindoleacetic acid (5-HIAA), the major serotonin metabolite.

The answer is D.

The levels of 5-HIAA in CSF correlate *inversely* with the frequency of aggression. Low level of 5-HIAA is associated with aggressive behavior and suicide through violent methods.

Neurotransmitters and aggression:

Induction of aggression: Dopamine.

Inhibition of aggression: Norepinephrine, serotonin, GABA.

54. To which ion channel is GABA functionally related?

A. Sodium.
B. Potassium.
C. Chloride.
D. Calcium.

The answer is C.

GABA is functionally related to chloride channels that are regulated by GABA and other ligands. When GABA binds to its receptors, the chloride channels open, allowing more chloride influx into the cell and therefore increasing membrane polarization. Benzodiazepines bind to specific sites on GABA receptors and facilitate the effects of GABA (increased affinity of the GABA receptors for GABA).

55. All of the following disorders are associated with unstable triplet (trinucleotide) repeat sequences EXCEPT:

A. Huntington's disease.
B. Fragile X syndrome.
C. Myotonic dystrophy.
D. Spinobulbar muscular atrophy.
E. Down's syndrome.

The answer is E.

Down's syndrome is trisomy 21, meaning that the patient has three replicates of chromosome 21, not a triplet repeat of nucleotides within a gene. All other conditions listed above are associated with unstable triplet repeat sequences.

56. What disorder in early life shows similar pathologic changes to those in Alzheimer's disease?

A. Fragile X syndrome.
B. Prader–Willi syndrome.
C. Down's syndrome.
D. Williams's syndrome.

The answer is C.

The answer is Down's syndrome. Both Alzheimer's disease and Down's syndrome are associated with defects in chromosome 21. Persons with Down's syndrome who survive to early adulthood may present with histopathologic changes that are typical in Alzheimer's disease (senile plaques and neurofibrillary tangles). There is also a clear familial association between the two diseases.

57. What is the pharmacologic treatment of choice for decreasing the craving for alcohol?

A. A benzodiazepine.
B. Naloxone.
C. Disulfiram.
D. Naltrexone.

The answer is D.

Objectives of pharmacologic treatment for alcoholism are to:

Reduce craving: Opioid antagonists (naltrexone, nalmefene), SSRIs (fluoxetine, citalopram), lithium, and bromocriptine.

Ease withdrawal: Benzodiazepines.

Create adverse conditioning: Disulfiram.

58. What is the mechanism of disulfiram to treat alcohol dependence?

A. Inhibiting central opiate receptors.
B. Augmenting GABA-mediated inhibition.
C. Increasing serum acetaldehyde levels.
D. Preventing the breakdown of ethanol in the blood.

The answer is C.

Disulfiram inhibits alcohol-degrading enzyme acetaldehyde dehydrogenase and therefore raises blood levels of acetaldehyde, which can produce tachycardia, dyspnea, nausea, and vomiting. Disulfiram also inhibits dopamine β-hydroxylase.

Clinical effects of disulfiram last for up to 2 weeks after the last dose.

59. Data suggesting that alcoholism may be hereditary are based on studies of:

A. Siblings.
B. Parents.
C. Second-degree relatives.
D. Heterozygous twins.
E. Adopted siblings.

The answer is E.

Hereditary grounds in alcoholism were supported by studies of adopted siblings. The famous Danish adoption studies of familial determinants of alcoholism demonstrated that biologic sons of alcoholic persons were at higher risk of alcoholism than were biologic sons of nonalcoholic persons.

60. For what is the CAGE questionnaire used to screen?

A. Cocaine abuse.
B. Alcohol dependence.
C. Major depression.
D. General anxiety disorder.

The answer is B.

The CAGE questionnaire is used to screen patients for alcoholism; its letters stand for:

Cut: Have you ever felt you should cut down on your drinking?

Annoyed: Have people annoyed you by criticizing your drinking?

Guilt: Have you ever felt guilty about your drinking?

Eye-opener: Have you ever taken a drink as your first act in the morning, to steady your nerves or get rid of a hangover?

61. A middle-aged chronic alcoholic male appears in the emergency room with disorientation and confusion. A neurologic examination shows ataxia and disconjugate eye movements. What is the diagnosis?

A. Bilateral subdural hematoma.
B. Wernicke's encephalopathy.
C. Delirium tremens.
D. Pernicious anemia.

The answer is B.

Wernicke's syndrome is a condition of acute onset and is completely reversible.

Korsakoff's syndrome is chronic, and only 20% of patients may recover.

Symptoms of Wernicke's syndrome (also called alcoholic encephalopathy) are:

• Ataxia.
• Confusion.
• Ophthalmoplegia (horizontal nystagmus, abducens paralysis, disconjugate eye movements, and gaze palsy).

Pathophysiology: Thiamine deficiency.

62. What is the maximum period for which cocaine can be detected in the urine?

A. Less than 6 hours.
B. Seven to 12 hours.
C. Two to 4 days.
D. One week.
E. Two weeks.

The answer is C.

Cocaine's metabolite, benzoylecgonine, can be detected in the urine 2 to 4 days after cocaine is used.

63. In the emergency room, a 25-year-old female says that she is suicidal. She has been using crack cocaine in the past 5 days and feels depressed. She says that she had feelings of helplessness, hopelessness, and fatigue, with decreased appetite. What is the diagnosis?

A. Major depression.
B. Withdrawal syndrome.
C. Borderline personality disorder.
D. Anxiety disorder.

The answer is B.

Substance withdrawal syndrome can occur within hours to days after heavy use of a substance. It can be accompanied by significant mood changes. The acute onset of dysphoria, increased appetite, fatigue, psychomotor retardation or agitation, and sleep abnormalities (dreams, insomnia, or hypersomnia) that have followed cocaine use in the case described here are consistent with cocaine withdrawal, which again is usually paralleled by mood changes.

64. All of the following are clinical features of lysergic acid diethylamide (LSD) intoxication EXCEPT:

A. Paranoid ideation.
B. Depersonalization.
C. Tremor.
D. Synesthesia.
E. Pupillary constriction.

The answer is E.

Behavioral changes: Fear, anxiety, paranoid ideation, impaired judgment.

Perceptual changes: Perceptual changes in full wakefulness, depersonalization, derealization, illusions/hallucinations, and synesthesias.

Other: Pupil dilation.

Synesthesia: A sensation or hallucination caused by another sensation.

65. Which of the following is the most popular addictive substance in the United States?

A. Nicotine.
B. Alcohol.
C. Cocaine.
D. Heroin.
E. PCP.

The answer is A.

The most popular addictive substance is nicotine.

Among all the substance addictions, addiction to nicotine contributes most to premature death and disability, and is associated with the highest annual mortality.

66. A 24-year-old male who is well-known as a drug abuser to the emergency room staff is brought in by police after being found in a disoriented and confused state in the street. Upon examination, you find that the patient has mildly enlarged pupils, marked diaphoresis, lacrimation, and muscle ache. He yawns constantly during the examination and states that he has abdominal discomfort. What is your preliminary diagnosis?

A. Cocaine intoxication.
B. Cocaine withdrawal.
C. PCP intoxication.
D. Opiate intoxication.
E. Opiate withdrawal.

The answer is E.

Opioid withdrawal symptoms include disorientation, confusion, dysphoric mood, increased muscle tone, mildly enlarged pupils, increased blood pressure and heart rate, marked diaphoresis, piloerection, lacrimation (or rhinorrhea) and salivation, nausea or vomiting, diarrhea, yawning, fever, and insomnia.

67. A 28-year-old male is seen in the emergency room. He is comatose, with pinpoint pupils and decreased respiratory effort. His urine drug screen is positive for opiate. What is the immediate treatment of choice?

A. IV dextrose.
B. IV thiamine.
C. IV naloxone.
D. IV flumazenil.

The answer is C.

This is a case of severe opioid intoxication.

Symptoms of opioid intoxication: Pupillary constriction with drowsiness or coma, slurred speech, impairment in attention or memory, and pulmonary edema from central respiratory inhibition.

The pupils may be dilated from anoxia due to severe overdose.

Treatment of opioid intoxication: Naloxone 0.4 mg IV for respiratory depression or stupor.

Treatment of withdrawal: Clonidine or methadone.

The other choices shown are not for opioid intoxication. IV dextrose is for hypoglycemia, IV thiamine is for Wernicke's syndrome, and IV flumazenil is for benzodiazepine intoxication.

68. Which of the following is not the clinical feature of PCP intoxication?

A. Nystagmus.
B. Hypotension or bradycardia.
C. Muscle rigidity.
D. Hyperacusis.
E. Numbness to pain.

The answer is B.

Signs of PCP intoxication:

1. Neurologic: Vertical or horizontal nystagmus, numbness, ataxia, dysarthria, muscle rigidity.
2. Autonomic: Hypertension, increased bronchial and salivary secretions.
3. Mental: Hyperacusis, labile affect, agitation, and assaultiveness.

PCP binds to N-methyl-D-aspartate subtype of glutamate receptors.

69. According to the *Diagnostic and Statistical Manual of the American Psychiatric Association, Fourth Revision* (DSM-IV), which of the following differentiates substance dependence from abuse?

A. Tolerance and withdrawal.
B. Social dysfunction.
C. A period of 12 months is required to make the diagnosis.
D. Interpersonal problems.

The answer is A.

The criteria for dependence include tolerance or withdrawal, which are not criteria for abuse.

70. What are the sleep abnormalities that may be detected with electroencephalography in depression?

A. Shortened latency of rapid-eye-movement (REM) sleep.
B. Decreased length of the first REM episode.
C. Decreased REM density.
D. Increased stage 4 sleep.

The answer is A.

In general, depressed patients have a reduced proportion of non-REM sleep and increased proportion of REM sleep.

1. Shortened REM latency.
2. Increased length of the first REM episode.
3. Increased REM density.
4. Decreased stage 4 sleep.
5. Increased awakening during the second half of the night.

71. All of the following are clinical features of post-traumatic stress disorder (PTSD) EXCEPT:

A. Re-experiencing of the event.
B. Increased arousal.
C. Avoidance of stimuli.
D. Duration of disturbance ranges from 1 week to 1 month.

The answer is D.

Key points in the diagnosis of PTSD:

Exposure to a traumatic event and:

Re-experiencing the event.

Increased arousal.

Avoidance of stimuli.

Numbing of general responsiveness.

Symptoms last longer than 1 month.

If the duration of the disturbance is less than 1 month, the disorder might be diagnosed as acute stress disorder.

72. All of the following diagnoses are categorized as somatoform disorders EXCEPT:

A. Briquet's disease.
B. Pain disorder.
C. Body-dysmorphic disorder.
D. Munchausen's syndrome.
E. Hypochondriasis.

The answer is D.

Munchausen's syndrome is a factitious disorder with predominately physical signs and symptoms. It is not included in the category of somatoform disorder.

DSM-IV includes seven diagnoses under the category of somatoform disorders:

Somatization disorder (also known as Briquet's syndrome), conversion disorder, hypochondriasis, pain disorder, body dysmorphic disorder, undifferentiated somatoform disorder, and somatoform disorder not otherwise specified.

73. The most common electrolyte imbalance seen in eating disorders is:

A. Hyponatremia.
B. Hypernatremia.
C. Hypokalemia.
D. Hyperkalemia.
E. Hypercalcemia.

The answer is C.

Hypokalemia.

When cardiac disturbance (anxiety, palpitation) is suspected in patients with an eating disorder, check the patient's serum potassium concentration.

74. A 30-year-old female was referred by her internist for a consultation. She has repetitively presented herself with abdominal crises, paresthesias, and weakness. She has also had anxiety of sudden onset with severe mood swings, as well as frequent angry outbursts, and has sometimes complained of hearing voices. Her routine work-up has been completely negative. Besides somatoform disorders, factitious disorders, and borderline personality disorders, what would you consider in your differential diagnosis?

A. Angina.
B. Acute intermittent porphyria.
C. Acute appendicitis.
D. Acute pancreatitis.

The answer is B.

Acute intermittent porphyria.

Symptoms: Colicky abdominal pain with nausea and vomiting, psychotic symptoms such as hallucinations, agitated depression, and polyneuropathy.

Acute intermittent porphyria has been estimated to be undiagnosed in 0.5% of psychiatric patients.

Test: Urine porphobilinogen and uroporphyrin.

75. A 30-year-old male presents with episodes of irresistible urges to sleep of sudden onset, and usually accompanied by a loss of muscle tone. It happened as often as four times a day and often lasts 10 to 20 minutes. The patient has also had vivid dreams while still conscious. What is the diagnosis?

A. Sleep terror.
B. Nightmare.
C. Narcolepsy.
D. Obstructive apnea.

The answer is C.

This is a typical case of narcolepsy. The DSM-IV criteria for this condition require that the episodes occur daily for more that 3 months, and present as one or both of the following:

1. Cataplexy (sudden loss of muscle tone, often precipitated by strong emotion), followed by entry into the REM stage of sleep within a few minutes of falling sleep;
2. Repeated intrusions of REM sleep into the transition between sleep and wakefulness (as manifested by hypnopompic or hypnagogic hallucinations or sleep paralysis).

Both nightmare disorder and sleep-terror disorder are parasomnias. Patients with nightmare disorder can remember the details of frightening dreams, whereas those with sleep-terror disorder cannot. In obstructive apnea, breathing is interrupted because of airway blockage (patients usually are obese), and respiratory effort continues.

76. Findings associated with diabetic neuropathy include all the following EXCEPT:

A. Numbness and pain.
B. Tremor.
C. Muscle weakness and atrophy.
D. Incontinence.
E. Postural hypotension.

The answer is B.

Diabetic neuropathy may present with sensory deficits (numbness and pain from mononeuropathy), autonomic neuropathy including incontinence, neurogenic bladder (with recurrent urinary tract infection), postural hypotension, and motor abnormalities that may result in muscle weakness and atrophy. Retinal and cranial-nerve involvement (oculomotor, trochlear, and abducens nerves) by mononeuropathy simplex are very common. However, diabetic neuropathy does not cause tremor.

77. A 78-year-old white male presents with a complaint of gradual deterioration in memory and ability to take care of his bank accounts. His caregiver reports that he also mumbles to himself, laughs, or yells for no reason, and easily becomes agitated. The patient's gait is impaired. He has been wheelchair-bound for the past 2 years. A computed tomographic scan of the head shows generalized atrophy. The patient's CSF shows 51 white blood cells (WBCs)/mm^3, of which 46 are lymphocytes. The CSF protein is 112 mg/dL. The γ-globulin concentration in the patient's CSF is elevated. Oligoclonal bands are present upon protein electrophoresis of the CSF. The most important next test is:

A. Immunoblot detection of PrP^{Sc}.
B. EEG.
C. MRI.
D. Fluorescent treponemal antibody absorption test (FTA-ABS).
E. CSF morphology.

The answer is D.

This is a typical case of late neurosyphilis, which presents with dementia and other psychiatric symptoms. The patient may also have both tabes dorsalis and taboparesis as the cause of his wheelchair-bound status. His CSF has an elevated WBC count (predominantly lymphocytes) and protein concentration, increased γ-globulin concentration, and presence of oligoclonal protein bands. The next test done should be a treponemal confirmatory test such as blood FTA-ABS or MHA-TP.

Immunoblot detection of PrP^{sc} is a test for Creutzfeldt–Jakob disease.

EEG and MRI are nonspecific for neurosyphilis.

Cerebrospinal fluid (CSF) morphology may be helpful for the diagnosis of lymphoma of the central nervous system (CNS), but not for neurosyphilis.

78. All of the following pathologic findings are characteristic of idiopathic Parkinson's disease EXCEPT:

A. Loss of pigmentation in the substantia nigra.
B. Neurofibrillary degeneration in the substantia nigra.
C. Cell loss in the substantia nigra.
D. Cell loss in the globus pallidus and putamen.
E. Presence of eosinophilic intraneural inclusion granules.

The answer is B.

The pathologic features of idiopathic parkinsonism include loss of pigmentation and cells in the substantia nigra and other brain-stem centers, cell loss in the globus pallidus and putamen, and the presence of eosinophilic intraneural inclusion granules (Lewy bodies) in the basal ganglia, brain stem, spinal cord, and sympathetic ganglia.

Neurofibrillary tangles as well as neuritic plaques and granulovacuolar degeneration are typical histopathologic features in Alzheimer's dementia.

79. A 25-year-old female complains of progressive numbness and weakness in the shoulders and arms. Physical examination shows deficient sensation of pain and temperature in the shoulders and both upper extremities. Touch and vibration sensations, however, are preserved. Deep tendon reflexes are absent. Muscle atrophy is noticed in the patient's forearms and hands. The most likely diagnosis can be confirmed by:

A. MRI.
B. Serum vitamin B$_{12}$ assay.
C. CSF examination.
D. Muscle biopsy.
E. Serum creatine phosphokinase (CPK) assay.

The answer is A.

This is a case of anterior spinal cord lesion. Possible etiologies include syringomyelia, spinal compression, and occlusion of the anterior spinal artery. Pain and temperature appreciation are impaired below the level of the lesion, by involvement of the lateral spinothalamic tract. In addition, weakness or paralysis of muscles supplied by the involved segments of the cord results from damage to motor neurons in the anterior horn. However, there is relative preservation of posterior column function such as the sensations of touch and vibration. The best procedure for viewing the spinal-cord pathology in such a case is MRI.

The symptoms do not indicate vitamin B$_{12}$ deficiency.

CSF examination may show nonspecific change, but is not helpful for locating a morphologic change in the cord.

Muscle biopsy and measurement of the serum CPK level are useful in diagnosing neuromyopathy.

80. A 41-year-old male complains of pain about the ear, difficulty in closing his right eye, and drooping of his right face. He finds that his right ear is very sensitive to loud, low-frequency sounds. When a small spoonful of sugar is applied to the right side of his tongue, he says that it tastes like sand. Physical examination shows right-sided weakness of both the upper and lower face. The patient's symptoms started 3 days ago. The most likely diagnosis is:

A. Stroke.
B. Diabetic neuropathy.
C. Chronic migraine.
D. Idiopathic Bell's palsy.
E. Tic douloureux.

The answer is D.

Bell's palsy is a facial weakness of the lower-motor-neuron type. It is caused by idiopathic facial-nerve involvement outside the CNS. Ear pain is common. Impairment of taste, lacrimation, or hyperacusis can also be present. The onset can be abrupt. The symptoms can progress in hours to a day.

The lower-motor-neuron symptom rules out stroke, which involves upper motor neurons in the CNS.

Diabetic neuropathy rarely involves the trigeminal nerve. There are no other symptoms in this case that indicate diabetic neuropathy.

Although chronic migraine can present with acute exacerbation, the clinical context of this case is not consistent with such a diagnosis.

Tic douloureux (trigeminal neuralgia) presents with typical pain in areas of the face supplied by the second and third divisions of the trigeminal nerve. No facial weakness is found on examination.

81. In radiologic examination of the brain, CT is preferred over MRI when:

A. A good differentiation of white from gray matter is essential.
B. The presumed lesion is in the posterior fossa or brain stem.
C. Acute hemorrhage is suspected.
D. The patient is pregnant.
E. The patient suffers from claustrophobia.

The answer is C.

Advantages of CT:

1. Detection of acute bleeding (less than 24 to 72 hours old).
2. Suitable for patients with metallic implant.
3. No need for a prolonged stay in a narrow space (which may induce claustrophobia).

Advantages of MRI:

1. Excellent soft-tissue contrast reveals white matter.
2. Excellent imaging of the posterior fossa and brain stem.
3. Preferable in pregnancy.

82. A positive Romberg's test indicates dysfunction of the:

A. Dorsal columns.
B. Cerebellar vermis.
C. Muscles of the lower extremities.
D. Vestibular system.
E. Vascular supply of the lower extremities.

The answer is A.

Neurologic tests:

Romberg's test: Dorsal-column function.
Stance and gait: Cerebellar-vermis function.
Muscle strength: Muscles of the lower extremities.
Nylen-Barany (Dix–Hallpike) maneuver: Vestibular-system function.
Doppler ultrasonography: Vascular supply of the lower extremities.

83. Characteristic clinical features and examination findings in cases of hypertensive encephalopathy include all of the following EXCEPT:

A. Headache and vomiting.
B. Seizures.
C. Papilledema, retinal arteriolar spasm, retinal hemorrhages, and exudates.
D. CT scan usually shows a normal brain.
E. MRI T2-weighted phase study shows low-density areas suggestive of edema.

The answer is D.

In hypertensive encephalopathy, both CT and T2-weighted MRI scans show low-density areas suggestive of edema in the posterior regions of hemispheric white matter.

84. Which of the following results of hearing assessment indicates conductive hearing loss:

A. Rinne's test: Air conduction as fast as bone conduction.
B. Weber's test: Sound perceived as coming from normal ear.
C. Weber's test: Sound perceived as coming from midline.
D. Weber's test: Sound perceived as coming from affected ear.
E. Rinne's test: Bone conduction slower than air conduction on affected side.

The answer is D.

Normal:

Weber's test: Sound perceived as coming from midline.

Rinne's test: Air conduction faster than bone conduction.

Sensorineural hearing loss:

Weber's test: Sound perceived as coming from normal ear.

Rinne's test: Air conduction faster than bone conduction.

Conductive hearing loss:

Weber's test: Sound perceived as coming from affected ear.

Rinne's test: Bone conduction faster than air conduction on affected side.

85. Clinical findings in myasthenia gravis include all of the following EXCEPT:

A. Slowly progressive course.
B. Diplopia, ptosis, dysarthria, and dysphagia.
C. The weakness does not conform to the distribution of any single nerve.
D. Pupillary responses are often affected.
E. Persistent activity of a muscle group leads to temporarily increased weakness, with restoration of strength after a brief rest.

The answer is D.

Myasthenia gravis affects neuromuscular transmission in skeletal muscle. The postsynaptic receptor involved in this process is a nicotinic-type acetylcholine receptor. Pupillary responses are instead controlled by the autonomic system. The postsynaptic receptor in the parasympathetic system is the muscarinic receptor, which differs from the nicotinic receptor, and the postsynaptic receptors in the sympathetic system are adrenoceptors. Thus, myasthenia gravis does not effect pupillary responses.

In Preparation for the Board: Practical Tips

Test taking is never a pleasant experience unless you are prepared to score high. Though a solid foundation of knowledge is essential, it does not guarantee success in an examination. Even master clinicians cannot always translate their expertise into a score compatible with their clinical competence. Many textbooks, comprehensive review books, audio/video tapes, and live lecture programs are available in psychiatry and neurology, and the majority of them provide fairly thorough coverage of the information required by the written examination of ABPN (the Board). Readers are encouraged to utilize these resources to build a strong knowledge base. There is no shortcut to learning psychiatry. However, for those who are already well-learned, proper preparation may reorganize their knowledge and put them into a test-ready status, and thereby substantially improve their score, in a short period of weeks or even days. This book is designed to help the organization of a thorough study as well as providing last-minute information for the ABPN examination. For the tedious task of preparing for the Board, we believe that providing intensive study for a period of at least 4 months is needed. The following is a suggested plan for such a 4-month study.

Four months before the ABPN examination, the first round of study (weeks 1 to 10): Strengthen vulnerable areas.

- Read *Psychiatry for the Boards*. This may help indicate the kind of material you will need.
- Collect and organize the necessary study material (see the book list that follows).
- Make a study plan for the following 10 weeks. You may want to digest several (3 to 5) intensive chapters in those areas in which your training program may have been relatively weak.

Remember that although many residency programs claim certain strengths in their training, the ABPN requires a "balanced" clinical knowledge and skill.
- Study every day. Daily study is proven to be superior to periodic rigorous "cramming."

Highlight your material. Make brief notes and use mnemonics.

Two months before the ABPN examination, the second round of study (weeks 11 to 14): Sharpen your learned knowledge.

- Answer the questions in this book.
- Reorganize your material. If there is any major area of material that you did not have time to digest in the previous 10 weeks, you will probably not be able to complete it. Do not attempt to do so; you will never be competent in every area of psychiatry. For passing the ABPN examination, you need only one thing: the total score.
- Plan your study for the next 4 weeks. It is essential to budget most of your time for reviewing those areas you already studied. Remember, in order to increase your score, you have to master the knowledge in a particular area, not merely acquaint yourself with it. Too often test-takers are frustrated when given a question that looks familiar but to which they cannot ascertain the right answer.
- Put aside a small amount of material that you need to read one more time before the examination.

Two weeks prior to the ABPN examination, the critical third round of study (weeks 15 to 16): This book should give you powerful support at this stage.

- Your extensive study may not translate into a high score on the ABPN examination until you read *Psychiatry for the Boards*. If you already read the book at the beginning of your 4-month study period, you should read it a second time now.

- Review highlighted or checked material. Time is ticking. Do not spend more time in learning any new topics, unless they are very short and you feel they are very important. Write down a few mnemonics (e.g., milestones of development).

Two days before the ABPN examination. Last minute cram.

Read *Psychiatry for the Boards* one more time. Review mnemonics.

The night before the ABPN examination. Do not study! You've done enough. You are ready for the examination.

- Engage in some light aerobic exercise.
- Listen to soothing music.
- Rest well and replenish your energy.

Suggestions for further reading:

Everyone has an individual style of studying. A good review book for the ABPN examination should match the scope of knowledge required by the Board, should have a reader-friendly format, and should be of a manageable size. Many of our colleagues found the following books particularly helpful, although not necessarily in the order shown (since this depends on the needs of your training program and your personal preferences).

1. Kaplan KI, Sadock BJ. *Synopsis of psychiatry*, 8th ed. Baltimore: Williams & Wilkins, 1998.
2. Kaplan KI, Sadock BJ. *Study guide and self-examination review for Kaplan & Sadock's Synopsis of Psychiatry*, 7th ed. Philadelphia: Lippincott Williams & Wilkins, 2000.
3. Arana GW, Rosenbaum JF. *Handbook of psychiatric drug therapy*, 4th ed. Philadelphia: Lippincott Williams & Wilkins, 2000.
4. Simon RP, Aminoff MJ, Greenberg DA. *Clinical neurology*, 4th ed. Stamford, CT: Appleton & Lange, 1999.
5. Stern TA, Herman JB. *Psychiatry update and Board preparation*, New York: McGraw Hill, 2000.

6. Kaufman DM. *Clinical neurology for psychiatrist,* Orlando: Harcourt Health Sciences Group, 2001.
7. Lieberman JA, Tasman A. *Psychiatric drugs,* Philadelphia: WB Saunders, 2000.
8. Stahl SM. *Psychopharmacology of antipsychotics,* London, UK: Dunitz, Martin Ltd., 1999.
9. Stahl SM. *Psychopharmacology of antidepressants,* London, UK: Taylor and Francis Books Ltd., 1997.
10. Simon RI. *Concise guide to psychiatry and law for clinicians*, Washington, DC: APP, 1998.

Subject Index